Dr Rosemary Leonard is one of the country's best-known doctors. She is the resident doctor on *BBC Breakfast*, and also writes for the *Daily Express* and *S* magazine, and is the medical editor for *Woman and Home* magazine. She also writes for MSN and myhealth.london.nhs websites.

Although she is a regular broadcaster, Rosemary is still very much a practising doctor, working as a part-time GP partner in a busy South London surgery, where she has a special interest in women's health. She trained in medicine at Cambridge University and St Thomas's Hospital Medical School. She has been the GP representative on the Committee on Safety of Medicines, a member of the Human Genetics Commission and a director of the Health Protection Agency. In 2004 Rosemary was awarded an MBE for her services to healthcare.

Rosemary lives with her husband and two sons and enjoys hiking, skiing, sailing and gardening. This is her third book.

You can find Dr Rosemary Leonard on Facebook, follow her on Twitter @DrRosemaryL or visit her web page www.drrosemaryleonard.co.uk.

Praise for *Doctor, Doctor*:

'A riveting read' *Daily Express*

'She has a breezy, confident style that makes this an entertaining glimpse into the sharp end of medicine' *The Lady*

'Funny, heartwarming – and you can skip the gory bits' *Yours*

DR ROSEMARY LEONARD

Doctor, Doctor

Incredible True Tales from a GP's Surgery

headline

The right of Rosemary Leonard to be identified as the Author of
the Work has been asserted by her in accordance with the
Copyright, Designs and Patents Act 1988.

First published in 2012
by HEADLINE PUBLISHING GROUP

This edition first published in 2013
by HEADLINE PUBLISHING GROUP

2

Cataloguing in Publication Data is available from the British Library

978 0 7553 6206 6

Typeset in Baskerville by Avon DataSet Ltd,
Bidford-on-Avon, Warwickshire

Printed and bound by CPI Group (UK) Ltd, Croydon, CR0 4YY

Headline's policy is to use papers that are natural, renewable and
recyclable products and made from wood grown in sustainable forests.
The logging and manufacturing processes are expected to conform to the
environmental regulations of the country of origin.

HEADLINE PUBLISHING GROUP
An Hachette UK Company
338 Euston Road
London NW1 3BH

www.headline.co.uk
www.hachette.co.uk

www.drrosemaryleonard.co.uk

AUTHOR'S NOTE

The essence of each of the stories in this book is based on my experience as a GP for twenty-three years. However, certain details have been altered and stories merged to protect the identities and confidentiality of patients and colleagues.

The exceptions to this are Gordon and Jack, who have given permission for their stories to be used. The story of my being taken hostage by a patient in Chapter 6, and the resulting court case, is all true; and it is also true that a patient made a complaint to the GMC similar to the story of Roger in Chapter 10.

CONTENTS

CHAPTER ONE

BACK TO THE BEGINNING

'So Rosemary, why do you want to become a doctor?'

It was 1973 and I had set my heart on gaining a place at Newnham College, Cambridge, to study medicine. This interview was crucial and I had anticipated the obvious question. As I composed myself, I noticed weak sun rays shining through the window in the book-lined study, illuminating dust flecks in the air. The forbidding-looking woman in the brown tweed suit on the other side of the desk, who held my future in her hands, looked vaguely bored, as if she had heard it all before. Her short grey hair was styled severely and she peered over the glasses perched half-way down her nose. She looked at my entrance examination papers that lay on her desk and I saw her shift in her seat, a sure sign that she wanted me to hurry up so she could leave. She wouldn't have heard an answer like mine before, though – it was time to wake her up and get her attention.

My passion for medicine arose from an event that happened when I was a small girl. It was a cold Wednesday lunchtime in February, I was nine years old and late for lunchtime recorder practice – yet again. Time-keeping, then and now, has never been one of my strong points.

I was a pupil at Gravel Hill Junior School and a member of the recorder group there.

The group met in the school's main building but I'd left my instrument in my classroom, which was a temporary hut down a long path at the edge of the playing field. I was always doing this and, scared of being on the receiving end of yet another ear-bashing, I dashed back to get it.

There were two classrooms in the prefabricated building, with a corridor in between them where we hung our coats. Funds for public buildings were in very short supply in the early sixties, and many schools, including mine, had expanded into temporary huts. The drama group had already begun rehearsing in the classroom opposite mine – I could hear the members reciting Shakespeare. The walls were paper thin, so sound-proofing was minimal and I was well aware that if I made any noise I'd be in even more trouble. Unfortunately, as I ran into my classroom at full pelt, a gust of wind caught the outside door behind me. There was a strict school rule, rigidly enforced, forbidding anyone to slam doors, so I lurched clumsily to catch it before it thudded shut. Though light, the door had a razor sharp edge and I was off balance. It acted like a guillotine and sliced through my left index finger.

I don't remember any pain, but when I freed my hand from the door I saw that it had amputated three-quarters of my fingertip and that my hand was dripping copious amounts of blood. Did I scream? I can't remember. But I suspect not because no one came to help from the drama group. Bleeding all the way back to the main building, supporting my finger and its dangling tip with my other hand, I managed to reach the first aid room. Only then did I pass out.

My next memory is of the powerful smell of what I now know is ether in the casualty room of the Chalfont's and Gerrards Cross Hospital, the nearby cottage hospital. This was 1966 and, in those days, minor emergencies were dealt with there by a duty GP. The nearest large casualty department was at Wexham Park, the district hospital fifteen miles away, but clearly my partially amputated finger did not count as a 'major' emergency.

My mother, Edna, had been called by the school and she sat beside me, murmuring words of calm reassurance, while I watched Dr Webber meticulously insert nine stitches into the finger to reattach the tip. A white-capped nursing sister was there, too, with a crisp, starched apron, holding my hand in place. I wasn't scared, though. I was fascinated.

I wasn't given a general anaesthetic, so Dr Webber must have given me a highly effective local one, because I didn't feel a thing. I cannot recall any pain, even in the days afterwards, but I still clearly retain the image of those nine stitches – a row of neat, little, black knots just beneath the nail and extending around the back of my finger.

It was only when I was learning surgical techniques myself many years later that I realised the care Dr Webber had taken to try to preserve a fully functioning finger. He didn't have the benefit of an operating microscope or the magnifying glasses that surgeons use today – just his eyes, a very steady hand, a curved needle and a length of silk.

Nowadays patients go home the same day as an operation like that but, back then, things were very different. I spent the next two weeks lying in a hospital bed working my way through the complete set of Arthur Ransome's *Swallows and Amazons* books. Every six hours on the dot – day and night – I was given penicillin injections. I may not remember any pain in my finger, but having my bottom treated like a pin cushion and being jabbed with a needle twenty-eight times a week was unforgettable. It hurt like hell.

I was due to sit the 11-plus examination a year early but the accident put paid to that. My mother was actually pleased that I would have to wait another year at primary school because, having a birthday in July, I was young for my year anyway.

4

I returned to school, my finger swathed in an enormous bandage, and was amazed to discover that my blood was still smeared on the classroom door and all down the path. I can still picture it to this day – strange the things you remember. It brought back unwelcome memories and made me feel uncomfortable. I hated looking at it. I didn't say anything for days – I felt I'd caused enough trouble – but when I finally told my parents they were furious and rang the school to complain. The blood was gone by the following day.

My fingertip had gone blue almost immediately after the accident, which I thought was due to bruising. But as the weeks went by and the dressing was changed, I noticed it was not returning to its healthy pink colour but was turning black instead. After a month, Dr Webber informed me that my fingertip had lost its blood supply and had turned gangrenous. There was nothing that could be done to save it. It needed to be removed. Though I feel now I should have been appalled at this suggestion, I wasn't. After four weeks of having my finger heavily bandaged I was relieved to hear something was going to be done and that I would be able to use my hand again soon. And the black finger tip – especially the nail – looked so ugly I was glad that I was going to be rid of it.

This time I was admitted to Mount Vernon Hospital, in central Buckinghamshire, which was the nearest specialist plastic surgery department. The plan was for a piece of skin to be removed from my buttock and used to rebuild some sort of tip, so the finger wouldn't look stumped and short.

It didn't quite work out that way. Though a large piece of skin was removed from my buttock, the surgeon wasn't able to use it to rebuild my finger. Instead, he shortened it some more to make it look neater. But I didn't care – in the sixties they hadn't perfected the art of anaesthetics and most people vomited for hours after being in theatre – and I was no exception. Immediately after the operation I forgot about my finger. All I cared about was stopping being sick and getting my head out of a bowl.

The bandages came off relatively quickly but my skinned bottom needed padding for two more months because the raw skin was still so painful. In retrospect it shouldn't have taken that long – I suspect that either the knife went too deep or it got infected. Embarrassingly, I had to sit on a cushion at school and was excused games and swimming. I suspect I capitalised on this at home. Like most couples at the time, my parents' discipline of choice was a well-delivered smack to my bottom. My bum, though, was safely off limits for now.

The treatment I had received at Mount Vernon had given me a ringside seat at one of the best hospitals in the country and sparked in me an interest in medicine. While I had been there, I had seen children with far more serious injuries than mine who had undergone very complex surgery. I marvelled at what doctors could do and became enthralled by the workings of the human body.

From then on I was determined to become a doctor and my ambition never wavered. According to my mother, I never remotely considered anything else and I picked my O and A levels with a medical career in mind. It was fortunate that I'd been good at science, especially as back then medicine was not a common choice of career for a woman. I still remember the careers teacher asking what I was going to when I didn't get into medical school. So much for positive encouragement. Luckily, though, there were other staff who were much more enlightened.

I'm a middle child. My elder sister Christine is two years older and Margaret, the baby of the family, is seven-and-a-half years younger. They are both taller than me, which they get from my father's side of the family. I'm short like my mother and I'm the one that most resembles her.

Christine is a real brain-box and was a very hard act to follow – she never got less than an A in anything she tackled. She went to Cambridge two years ahead of me, where she got a triple first – a first in all three end of year exams. She's now a professor in molecular parasitology at Heidelberg University in Germany. Margaret is a dentist and trained at Bristol.

Home was in Chalfont St Peter, South Buckinghamshire, where we lived in a four-bedroom detached house on a hillside that was bought from new in 1961. It was a typical early-sixties family house with a reasonable-sized back garden which was about fifty feet square. My parents moved there from the London suburb of Ealing when I was five for a better quality of life, though I don't think it improved life for my father, Gordon. He then had a long commute along Western Avenue to Acton in west London where he worked as an engineer for a large company that made engine components for cars, buses and trucks.

I don't think my parents were aware of the fact before we moved but South Bucks had – and continues to have – fantastic state schools. I started at Dr Challoner's High School, one of the best girls' grammars in the country, a year after my accident, and I'm convinced it was the quality of my education there that enabled me to strive for Cambridge, despite the negative remarks from the careers teacher! Sibling rivalry played a role, too – if my older sister could get in, then so could I.

Back in 1974, Cambridge was a very male-dominated establishment. Only six colleges offered places for women – three of these were mixed and, though I would have loved to have gone to a college where there were men as well as women, they only had five places each for women studying medicine. At the women-only colleges, there were up to ten places – so I stood a much better chance of getting in there. Newnham was the nearest one to the centre of town and, of course, I knew of it because my sister was already there.

I had a wonderful three years in Cambridge. I had to work incredibly hard – medicine is a tough option with a full timetable – but I managed to find time to play hard as well. And, though I was in a women-only college, the rules about visitors were very liberal, and with a heady ratio of seven men to each woman in the university, I didn't lack male company. I had no idea back then that I would end up working as a medical journalist for the BBC, and be required to give expert comments on a wide range of different topics. Many of the medical contacts I now use for professional advice on stories I cover are friends I first got to know in my student days nearly thirty years ago.

I can't remember what it's like to have two complete hands because it happened so long ago. At the age of nine the only adjustment I had to make was to stop learning to play the oboe because my short finger couldn't reach the top key, but I continued to play the piano. However, I would always be rubbish at scales. You need even pressure on all ten digits and regular rhythm, and that was never going to happen with my stump. It always seemed to land on the keys out of time and with a bump.

The only lasting problem I've had has been extreme sensitivity to cold in the short tip, which made playing hockey at school in the winter a complete misery. I quickly learnt that mittens are warmer than gloves, and wearing two pairs means I can enjoy skiing. I also take particular care to hide the finger when I'm demonstrating anything on TV because I feel viewers could be distracted by its strange appearance. Surprisingly, there have been times when my foreshortened finger has come in useful, especially when treating patients with minor disfigurements.

I'd known eighteen-year-old Emma since her mum brought her in for her six-week-old baby check-up. She'd always suffered from mild eczema and I still saw her at least twice a year to discuss how to manage it. On one occasion in her early teens she had come in with very puffy eyes from an allergic reaction to mascara and we'd had frequent discussions about which brand of make-up was likely to suit her best. My skin is sensitive, too, though not as bad as hers, and I'd learnt the hard way from the BBC and other make-up rooms that some brands were more likely to irritate than others.

When I saw her name on my list one early summer morning I assumed more of the same. But instead of a lively, happy teenager walking through the door, my first sight of Emma was a glittery pink sock covering a left foot, followed by a horizontal leg in a bright pink plaster cast. Finally the rest of Emma emerged. She was in a wheel-chair, which was being ineptly pushed by her mother, Susan, who wedged one of the wheels against the door frame as she came in. Emma winced. Susan reversed, realigned, came in successfully but knocked over my bin with Emma's plaster cast. Her daughter winced again. If I hadn't been there, I suspect there would have been some ripe swearing – from both the driver and the passenger.

The broken leg wasn't the whole picture. Emma had clearly been in an accident and her left arm was also encased in pink plaster that extended from her biceps to her fingers. While the wheelchair was being manoeuvred, I had a quick look at her records to see if any letters had arrived from a hospital with details of what had happened. Nothing – which didn't surprise me. If often takes weeks for letters to arrive. So I had to ask Emma to fill me in. Apart from her eczema, she had never had any medical problems and she came from a sporty family – her father had been a competitive cyclist before he snapped his Achilles tendon and had to ride more cautiously. Like her father, Emma was a keen cyclist, too.

'Hello, Emma,' I said. 'What on earth has happened to you?'

'Quite a lot unfortunately,' said Emma. 'I was out cycling with friends on a country road in Kent when some idiot car driver hit my bike and I ended up smashing into a telegraph pole.'

'How dreadful,' I said. 'I hope the driver stopped to help?'

Her mother sighed, 'No – it was a classic hit and run. Whoever it was just drove off. No one has come forward to take the blame and whoever the low-life is, he or she just left my daughter unconscious against that pole without checking to see if she was OK. She could have been dead for all they cared.' Her eyes filled with tears.

'But I'm not dead, mum – my friends were there . . .'

'Thank goodness.'

'And the worst is over,' Emma consoled her, patting her mother's knee. 'Just concentrate on driving my wheelchair a bit better if you want me to live, OK?'

Her mother managed a weak smile.

'I can't recall any details about the car or its driver,' continued Emma. 'And though one of my friends knows it was a black BMW, that's the only details we have. The last thing I do remember is cycling round a particularly nasty bend in the road and wondering whether I could make it without using the brakes – I was going pretty fast.

'I reckon the car driver was caught unawares by the severity of the bend, too. He or she had probably underestimated it and had come round too fast and too tight, saw me too late and clipped my back wheel. My friends tell me I somersaulted off the bike before I hit the pole. My bike's a write-off.'

As well as injuring her left arm, leg and hand, Emma had hit her head, too. 'Wearing your cycling helmet probably saved your life,' I told her.

'I know,' said Emma. 'I used to hate wearing it when I was young because I thought it made me look like a jerk.'

'We'd have lots of rows about it,' said Susan, 'but I made it a rule: if Emma did not wear a helmet, then she was not allowed to ride her bike.'

'When I think of how I kicked up about that,' said Emma. 'As I got older, though, it had become a habit, thanks to mum, and I wouldn't dream of riding my bike with nothing to protect my head today, especially at the speeds I go now.'

Emma had also fractured her tibia and fibula (the lower leg bones), smashed her elbow to smithereens and broken her wrist.

I went through the list of injuries with her and delivered the bad news.

'I'm afraid that you won't be getting back on your bike for some time, Emma,' I told her. 'It is going to take a while for your leg and elbow to heal.'

She was going to be in plaster for at least another couple of months and would need intensive physiotherapy before she would be able to walk properly again or regain full use of her left arm. It was a small mercy that she was right-handed.

Emma was remarkably upbeat about it all. She didn't seem daunted by the long-haul treatment ahead and was confident that she would be back on her bike within a year.

'The hospital have been fantastic. I know everyone complains about the NHS but, honestly, I couldn't have asked for better treatment. The doctors and physios have been really lovely.' It was good to hear words of praise instead of the more common complaints.

Then, inexplicably, her mood changed and she dissolved into tears.

I offered Emma a tissue and told her it was perfectly normal to feel upset at having her life disrupted for so long.

'You don't understand,' she sniffed. 'It's not those injuries we've talked about that are upsetting me. I know you're going to think this is really stupid, Dr Rosemary, but I'm not worried about my broken bones, it's my hand. There's an injury there that is permanent and it is never going to heal. It's a life sentence.' It was only then I noticed that the middle finger of her left hand was swathed in its own large bandage and was clearly shorter than the others.

'Is some of your finger missing?' I asked.

A fresh bout of sobbing and half a box of tissues later, Emma composed herself enough to say, 'Yes, half of it, from the middle joint upwards. It looks so awful and disgusting. I'll never be able to wear nail polish again, people will stare and I'll feel a complete freak.' Emma said she had no idea what had happened to her fingertip. Apparently it had not arrived at the A&E department with the rest of her.

I asked to have a look and when I removed the bandage I saw that the hospital doctors had made a good job of sewing up the finger. It now ended at the second joint but looked as though it was healing well.

I put my own hands flat on the table and Emma glanced at them briefly before lifting her eyes to my face again. 'I'm going to have to live the whole of my life with a really ugly finger,' she said. 'People are going to stare and they will be horrified. It's gross.'

'I know it may seem awful now but it's really not the

end of the world,' I told her. 'You'd be amazed – people simply don't notice.'

'That's easy for you to say,' Emma said, blowing her nose. 'It will be so obvious and so embarrassing and no one will ever want to go out on a date with me. I'll probably never get married and have children. This has ruined my life.' She began crying again.

I began tapping the fingers of my left hand on the desk. Emma looked down at them and frowned, irritated by the noise. Still, she said nothing. I put my left hand up to my hair and brushed it back theatrically while she watched, then returned my hands to the desk with a thump.

'Look at my hands, Emma,' I said at last, exasperated. She did, but even then it took her some time to register my missing fingertip. When she did she gasped and put her good hand to her mouth and blushed.

'You have been seeing me, on average, twice a year since you were a baby,' I continued. 'I've held a stethoscope to your chest, given you jabs, held your hand, discussed make-up, but you've never noticed. Even now, when fingers are very much on your mind, you didn't see that a chunk of my left index finger is missing.'

'I feel so embarrassed,' whispered Emma. 'I should have noticed before.'

'Don't be,' I said. 'Honestly. I don't think people do notice, and if they do, they don't say anything. I don't think of myself as a freak and you're not one either. And as for attracting the opposite sex, you can cross that off your worry list. I've been married and I've had plenty of boyfriends and if they have even noticed my finger, they haven't cared. This will only change your life if you let it and you are a much stronger person than that.'

She didn't seem convinced. Though I knew the ortho-paedic specialists would look after her broken bones, I was concerned about her mental state and arranged to see her again the following week. I reminded myself that though I was quite used to my shortened finger, I'd had my accident when I was a child and, unlike Emma, I'd never had beautiful hands.

Not only that, but no matter how much she said she wasn't bothered by her other injuries, she was used to leading a very active lifestyle. Being immobilised by plaster would mean she would have a lot of time to think about her finger. After what she had been through it would be normal for her to become mildly depressed, but I was worried her low mood might become more severe.

The following week, her mother's wheelchair driving had improved, and this time she negotiated the doorway without removing any paintwork.

'How are you?' I asked.

'Oh, I'm fine.'

'Really?'

'Well, OK, then, I'm a bit fed up. No, that's wrong – I'm very fed up. I'm not good at sitting still. I think I'm getting on Mum's nerves.'

There was a nod from the other side of the room.

'And I'm worried I'm going to put on weight – what with no exercise and eating out of boredom. Thank goodness I'd finished my exams before this happened, but I've had to cancel all my plans for going travelling before I go off to uni.' She pulled a face.

'But,' she continued, 'before you ask, I'm not depressed. Honest. I'll get over all of this. I've just got to work out what I'm going to do for the next few months. I was thinking of doing some writing – I can manage to tap a keyboard with one-and-a-bit hands.'

It sounded like a good idea.

'Dr Rosemary,' she continued, 'can I ask you a personal question? You don't have to answer, of course, but I've seen you on TV and read some of your columns in news-papers and magazines. I wondered how you got into journalism and the media? Only, with all this time on my hands, I've started thinking about my career options.'

I was able to reassure her that it was a question I was frequently asked, and that I was more than happy to answer.

'It all happened by chance. After I qualified I was planning on a career in obstetrics and gynaecology, so I spent eight years training in that. But then I got married, and I realised that spending every third night and every third weekend on call in the hospital – which is what junior doctors had to do then – wasn't good for family life, especially once I had children. So I switched to general practice. I've been a GP round here since 1989. Soon after

I started, one of my patients was working on a new women's magazine – *Me* magazine – and asked me to write a weekly column on women's health – period pains, infertility problems, that kind of thing. I did that for eight years until the editor of *Me* moved to be Women's Editor of *The Sun* newspaper and she asked me to go with her. I started off just writing on women's health, as before, but then the news journalists asked me to comment on other health stories as well. Once my name was appearing regularly in *The Sun*, I started being asked to appear on TV programmes. I didn't have the expertise to deal with the media requests that were coming my way, so I signed up with an agent. One day she got a call asking for a doctor to appear on *BBC Breakfast* to talk about a new drug – Viagra. I'll always remember it – being a woman doctor talking openly about such a revolutionary new drug for men. That was fourteen years ago.'

'What about media training?' asked Emma. 'And your finger? Wasn't that a problem?'

'I've never done any formal training, but I've had lots of training on the job – if I made a hash of something, or wore something that didn't suit me, then someone at the BBC would tell me,' I explained. 'And, as for my finger, do you know – I'm not sure anyone at the BBC has ever noticed it – and if they have, they've never said a word to me. It really, really doesn't matter. I don't suppose I could do *Blue Peter* and demonstrate things with sticky back plastic, though . . .'

'Can I have another look at it?' Emma requested.

'Of course.'

I splayed my hands out on the desk and realised, with some horror, that they were not exactly in good condition. In fact, they looked awful. Gardening, my favourite hobby, had taken its toll. My nails were chipped and the skin was dry and rough. I apologetically admitted I had never paid that much attention to my hands.

'Do you think that's a legacy from the accident?' Emma asked shrewdly.

'Probably,' I admitted.

'Do you know, when the bandages come off, I don't think my finger is going to be that much shorter than yours,' she admitted. 'I've got to stop being so negative about this, haven't I? It really won't be so bad.'

That sounded better, but I still felt I needed to keep an eye on her and so I asked her to come back in a couple of weeks. By the time she did, her arm plaster was off and she managed to hobble in on crutches.

'I'm making progress,' she commented, 'and it's such a relief to be able to get around on my own. I feel a whole lot better not being reliant on Mum but, talking of her, both of us wanted me to ask you something. Have you ever had a manicure – you know, a proper professional manicure?'

'Never,' I admitted. 'As you noticed, I've always kind-of ignored my hands. I've never wanted to draw attention to them – because of my finger, I suppose. Ingrained in me since childhood. I paint my toenails, but I never paint my fingernails.'

She smiled.

A week later, a stiff cream envelope arrived at the surgery marked for my personal attention. It looked like an invitation of some sort.

But it wasn't. Instead it contained a gift card for the local beauty salon to have a manicure. The card read: 'With grateful thanks for all your help through the years. From the other "nine nails".'

It was one of the most thoughtful gifts I have ever received. And also one of the most expensive, because I've now become rather fond of treating my hands, cuticles and nails to some professional care. I stick to nude colours – I haven't quite had the nerve to paint them a trendy dark red, but maybe one day . . .

CHAPTER TWO

EXPRESS DELIVERY

I was having a heavy morning at the surgery and by 10am I badly needed some caffeine and a few minutes' relaxation before I saw my next patient. Just as I was about to go AWOL, Doreen Brown, our senior receptionist, rang me. We keep phone interruptions during surgery to a minimum, so I knew it had to be important and realised reluctantly that the coffee would probably have to wait.

'Sorry to bother you, Rosemary, but one of the patients waiting to see you is behaving very strangely,' Doreen told me. 'She's come in complaining of a tummy ache but one moment she's sitting quietly filling her face with junk food, and the next moment she's screaming and swearing. Could you see her urgently? I don't think we can leave her in the waiting room considering the state she's in. The other patients are getting twitchy.'

Josie waddled into my consulting room clutching a bag of chips in one chubby hand. She was mechanically shovelling fries into her mouth so fast that she clearly wasn't even going to stop to say hello. She did not look as though she was in pain so I was puzzled by what Doreen had said and felt a bit irritated. Doreen didn't usually make mistakes like this.

I thought longingly of the coffee I had missed while I gave this patient, whom I'd never seen before, the once-over. She fell heavily into the chair opposite and continued to eat – which was against the surgery rules and also, I thought, rather rude. I didn't want my room to smell of chips for the rest of the day, but telling her that wouldn't exactly start the consultation off very well so, unlike her, I kept my mouth shut. Josie was dressed in an over-sized grey tracksuit which failed to disguise the fact that she was very overweight. Her long hair was carelessly scraped back into a high ponytail that clearly demonstra-ted its two colours – two inches of dark roots and dry bleached ends. It was held in a scrunch band and she wore inch-long false nails.

I waited until she had finished the bag of chips, licked her fingers and wiped her greasy hands on her tracksuit bottoms. She beamed at me and her smile lit up the room. Underneath all that fat she was actually very pretty. 'Sorry,' she said, balling up the bag and throwing it in my bin. 'I can't seem to stop eating.' No wonder she has a stomach-ache when she eats that many chips so fast, I thought.

'Hello, I'm Dr Leonard, I don't think we've met before. The receptionist tells me you've been having tummy pains. When did they start and have you been sick as well?'

'No, I haven't thrown up,' she replied. 'I've had tummy aches before but nothing like this. It woke me up early this morning, it was so bad. I thought it might be wind and that if I ate something and went to the loo it would go away, but it didn't. I sat on the bog for half an hour but I couldn't go and the pain got worse. I'm worried I've got a blockage.'

Suddenly Josie's face and demeanour changed completely. Her face contorted in agony and she doubled over screaming, her arms crossed over her tummy. Tears spilled from her eyes and her back arched as waves of pain engulfed her. No way was she faking this and I rushed around the desk to massage her shoulders and whisper words of reassurance.

'Help me, help me, doctor, I can't bear it,' she yelled and rolled off the chair on to the floor where she curled up sobbing.

My initial thoughts were that Josie's bowel may have twisted. But why hadn't she vomited and how come she could still pig out on chips? I needed to examine her tummy but I couldn't persuade her to get off the floor. Crouching down, I gently pulled up her tracksuit top and my eyes must have widened in astonishment. It immediately became apparent that it wasn't just fat making Josie's stomach appear large. She was very, very pregnant and, I suspected, now in the throes of labour.

I held Josie's hand and waited for the pain to subside, then helped her on to the couch where I could examine her belly more carefully. I could feel the swelling of her womb, right up to the bottom of her breast bone, and I prodded carefully to try to ascertain how the baby was lying. It went through my mind like a blind flash of panic that there might be more than one baby, so I was hugely relieved to discover just one firm little bottom on the right below Josie's ribs. Good. That meant the baby was in the normal, head-down position at least.

I reached for my Pinard stethoscope, a funnel-like metal tube used to check a baby's heartbeat while it is in the womb. Pressing it gently on Josie's lower tummy, with the other end to my ear, I could clearly hear the unmistakable sound of a baby's heart, going at a healthy speed of around 120 beats a minute. There was no doubt about it.

'Josie, you are in labour,' I told her.

'What do you mean, in labour?' she asked. 'What does that mean? Is there something wrong with my guts?'

'No, Josie, you are about to have a baby.'

'What baby? I ain't got no baby. I ain't pregnant. I can't be.'

At that moment the next contraction started. Josie squeezed my hand so hard that her long, acrylic nails dug into my palm. As she screamed in agony I was tempted to join her because she had drawn blood.

I'd spent almost a decade training in obstetrics and gynaecology, and had delivered hundreds of babies. But

I'd always had the luxury of being in a hospital with everything I needed to hand – high-tech machinery, sterile instruments and a fully trained midwife. This was very different. Would I find myself tying an umbilical cord with a piece of string for the first time in my life?

My brain was racing. Josie was in complete denial about her pregnancy but that wasn't the issue. Could she give birth at any minute? Did we have the necessary equipment in the surgery? I needed to know how far advanced her labour was. I had to carry out a sterile vaginal examination because that is the only way to tell for sure. Working between contractions, I felt inside and judged that Josie's cervix was about six to seven centimetres dilated, which meant she was just over half-way through the first stage of labour. With luck she could get to hospital in time for the birth, but it might be touch and go. I phoned Doreen, explained the situation and asked her to arrange an ambulance as quickly as possible.

I also buzzed through to the practice nurse, Fiona O'Malley.

'Fi,' I said rather breathlessly, 'I've got a woman in labour – can you come and help me?'

'Sure, Rosemary, be with you in a second,' said Fiona calmly, as if this were the most natural request in the world.

Her voice was like balm and her reaction typical. Fiona is amazingly calm, no matter what she is faced with and if I were washed up on a desert island and could pick just one person to go with me it would be her. She's fearless, resourceful and a natural problem solver – one of those rare types who just gets on with it, instead of having hysterics.

Fiona arrived almost immediately, introduced herself to Josie and began speaking to her soothingly. Between contractions, we gently questioned Josie about the past nine months. I found it hard to believe she had never suspected she was pregnant, especially given my own experiences.

I gave birth to my elder son Thomas in 1989 and suffered pre-eclampsia during the pregnancy. This condition, which usually starts after the twentieth week, can cause complications for both mother and baby and affects between two and eight pregnant women in one hundred. It causes high blood pressure and protein leaks from the kidneys. If it's not picked up – and it usually is when protein is detected in the urine – a life-threatening condition called eclampsia – a type of seizure – can occur. It's now thought that pre-eclampsia occurs because of a problem with the placenta, but the only certain cure is to give birth.

Thomas was born by forceps delivery, aptly enough, at St Thomas's Hospital in Westminster, where I did my clinical training.

Pre-eclampsia usually happens only with the first baby and is rare in subsequent pregnancies, but I wasn't destined to have it easy when it came to motherhood.

When I was expecting William two years later, I developed severe pre-eclampsia, had to go off sick with a raging headache at 33 weeks and was immediately hospital-ised. William was born at 34 weeks and weighed only 2.2kg, which is less than 5 pounds. It was tough trying to get this tiny boy to feed during those first fraught few weeks but I did manage to do so eventually. I breastfed both sons for a year, despite having a mere thirteen weeks maternity leave and being back at work, along with night visits, when they were both three months old. It was a monumental juggling act and I'd express milk during my lunch break, feeling very much like a mechanical cow. I was also extremely tired, so I have a lot of sympathy for women embarking on the double tour de force of motherhood and work.

Yet here was Josie who had experienced none of the complications of pregnancy, despite having no medical care. She had sailed through it, totally unaware that she was going to become a mother.

Fiona asked her: 'Didn't you realise you were pregnant when your periods stopped?'

'No,' said Josie. 'I've never been regular and sometimes I go for months without having one. It was just normal for me.' Her face screwed up as another contraction contorted her body. By now I was keeping my hands well out of her way but Josie grabbed one of Fiona's instead.

'You didn't keep a diary of when the last one was?' asked Fiona through gritted teeth. It was only after the labour pain had subsided that she managed to extract her hand.

'No, I never.'

'Do you have a partner?' continued Fiona. 'We can ring him if you like; perhaps you would like him with you?'

Josie contracted again. This time we both kept our hands well out of the way. Instead I checked the baby's heart rate. It's normal for it to fall slightly during each contraction, but it should pick up again immediately afterwards. If it stayed low, it can be a sign that the baby is distressed.

'No, I don't have a bloke,' managed Josie eventually.

'But you must have had sex,' continued Fiona. 'The baby didn't get inside you without a man's help.'

'I met someone on holiday last year and we did it a few times, that's all,' said Josie. 'We didn't do it much, though; not enough to make a baby.'

Fiona and I widened our eyes at each other over Josie's contracting stomach. Young people today are bombarded by information about sex, and given sex education at school, and yet this poor almost-child, who was about to become a mum, was pitifully ignorant. Josie told us that she had never used contraception because she thought that if she didn't have monthly periods she couldn't get pregnant. To be fair to her, I'd heard this type of story many times before – that you needed to have sex more than once to conceive and that having erratic periods meant you were infertile. This was probably not the best time to dish out basic facts about sex but, between Josie's labour pains, Fiona and I tried to put her right about a few things, hoping words like 'once is enough', and 'protecting yourself' might take root.

'Didn't you suspect you were pregnant when your waist got bigger and your breasts became tender?' I asked.

'I knew I'd got fat,' said Josie; 'of course I did. But I always seemed so crazy to eat chocolate, 'specially chips, all the time, so I put it down to that. I never used to be heavy – this time last year I was a size twelve.'

Maybe I'd been unfair to Josie, I mused. Eating chips had perhaps been a pregnancy craving. I thought back to my own pregnancies. Both times I was aware, almost before I'd missed a period, that something was different. Luckily, I'd never been sick but I'd had moments when I felt nauseous. The most obvious sign had been a monumental, crashing tiredness that had me falling into bed, exhausted, at 8pm every night. This exhaustion had started in the first few weeks and carried on until the fourth month.

Although I hadn't craved chips, my must-have food – and I'd have virtually killed to get them – were jelly babies. Unsurprisingly, I was on the receiving end of many jokes about the psychological significance of this, but I didn't care about the baby shape of the sweets, it was their taste and texture I needed. The newsagent next to the surgery was so concerned about the effect of all that sugar sloshing around my teeth and rotting them that he rationed me to one large box a day, which I kept in the top drawer of my desk. I still like jelly babies but it was only in pregnancy that I just *had* to have them.

There are reported cases of 'concealed pregnancies' in medical literature, but until I met Josie I'd never quite bought the idea. No matter what a woman says, or wants to believe, surely deep down she knows? How could you *not* realise that your body was changing so dramatically? And how could you *not* feel your baby moving?

The latest contraction had finished, Josie was drained of colour and looked at me with large, scared eyes which bulged with tears. 'Are you sure I'm pregnant, doctor?' she whispered. 'Only, I told my mum I was just popping out for a loaf of bread.'

Fiona and I had to turn our faces away, finding it hard not to burst out laughing. This, after all, was a very different type of bun in the oven.

News of the birth drama in my consulting room spread fast. Doreen had rummaged around in the stockroom and miraculously appeared with a sterile delivery pack. I had the basic instruments I needed, including a proper cord clamp, should the baby decide to make a faster entry into the world than expected – and I had Fiona's help. That made me feel a lot more comfortable, especially as Josie's contractions were now coming at two-minute intervals. Where was the bloody ambulance? I phoned through to Doreen who said she would check that it really was on its way.

'Doctor, I need to go to the toilet to do a number two,' said Josie. Because she hadn't been to ante-natal classes,

Josie had no idea that the pressure in her pelvis and the pushing sensation in fact meant that she had reached stage two of labour. Fiona and I now knew that Josie would not be going anywhere. The baby was going to be born here.

I carried out an internal examination which confirmed that Josie's cervix was now fully dilated. Many women have tales of a hellish twenty-four hours of labour, but it seemed as if Josie's would be a maximum of six hours from that first morning tummy ache that had woken her.

I had to think fast and make a decision, even though common sense told me there wasn't one to make. Even if the ambulance arrived now it would be too late. It would be better for Josie and her baby if she gave birth in my room with a doctor and nurse present than in the back of an ambulance on the traffic-clogged roads of south London.

Despite my training, anxiety and fear had made my pulse rate rise and I could feel sweat collecting on my forehead and palms. I didn't want Josie to see how edgy I was, so I hid my nerves and tried to act as if I was calm and completely in control.

Fiona and I prepared a trolley. I washed my hands and put on sterile gloves. We explained to Josie that she had to obey our instructions.

Josie screamed loudly with every contraction and the air turned blue with her ripe language. The patients in the waiting room could have been left in no doubt about what was happening.

Fiona tried her best to calm Josie, who continued to swear and scream in pain.

'You pair of bloody cows,' she screamed. 'You've done nothing to stop the agony I'm in. I'm going home – you can't stop me. I've had enough of this.'

We didn't engage in any pointless dialogue but instead encouraged Josie to push hard. Soon we could see a small area of the baby's head, covered in pale hair, at the entrance of her vagina. Fiona stroked Josie's head, moistened her dry lips and spoke soothingly to her. 'You're nearly there,' she coaxed. 'Not long now, you're doing really well. Just try to relax between pushes . . .'

Josie then attempted to attack Fiona while trying to leave the couch and had to be eased back firmly.

'You bitches – you don't know what this is like,' screeched Josie.

'We do,' said Fiona sharply. 'Rosemary and I have had four babies between us and we have both delivered hundreds more, so just be a good girl and do exactly as we say.'

I told Josie to push less powerfully now that the birth was imminent so that the baby could be delivered in a controlled, gentle way that would minimise damage to vaginal tissue. But there was no chance of that. Josie was in total panic, tears streaming down her face, pushing and screaming and completely unable to hold back. It was one of the worst deliveries I have ever experienced. Fiona mopped Josie's brow and tried to calm her down, but it was useless and she smacked Fiona's hand away.

'I'll never forgive you for this,' Josie told us as another huge push took hold.

And this was the one that delivered the baby. However, instead of falling gently into my hands, like they say in the books, the infant shot from Josie's vagina like a bullet from a gun and I had to do a rugby dive to catch it. The beautiful little girl had just taken her first, deep breath, followed by the most almighty wail, when Doreen buzzed through that the ambulance crew had arrived. This newborn was destined to be a drama queen.

With a huge sigh of relief, I clamped and cut the umbilical cord, wrapped the infant in a blanket and placed her on Josie's tummy. She looked to be about 3kg and completely healthy. Josie was now silent. She was still in such complete shock that we feared she might drop her new daughter, so Fiona held the baby girl up to her mum so they could get a close look at each other.

Josie, the screaming banshee of a few minutes earlier, seemed to have left the room. I could even hear the clock ticking. The new mum regarded her baby in mute wonder. 'Has this come out of me? Is she mine?' Josie finally asked us in a reverential whisper.

I held her hand, 'You have a really beautiful daughter, Josie. But, before we do anything else, we need to get the afterbirth out.'

'Afterbirth, what's that?' The look of panic in her eyes had returned.

I explained it was a large cushion of tissue that fed the

baby while it was growing inside her. Josie regarded me through narrowed eyes, deeply suspicious.

Usually the mother is given a small injection in her bottom as the baby is being born, which helps the womb contract and expel the placenta. Because we hadn't got that drug in the surgery, I had to use the old-fashioned method of rubbing the uterus – not easy through Josie's many layers of fat. Even when the injection is given, the placenta can still get stuck and sometimes only half of it comes away. It was tempting to pull on the remains of the umbilical cord to get the job done quickly, but I needed to be patient and wait for placenta to separate naturally. Suddenly Josie yelled out again.

'Oh no, I've got another pain,' she screamed. 'There's another baby in there, isn't there? You cow, you didn't tell me that.'

I was fairly sure Josie's womb contained only a placenta but, even so, it was my turn to have a moment of panic, which Fiona detected. She felt Josie's tummy and gave me a pat of reassurance, too.

'No Josie, it really is just the afterbirth,' Fiona told her. 'Just give a little push to help Dr Leonard get it out.'

'Little push' was not something Josie understood. She pushed so hard that the placenta shot out across the couch and fell straight through my slippery hands on to the floor. Awful to admit, but it was difficult not to giggle because this was turning into a textbook case of 'how not to deliver a baby'.

I surveyed the aftermath. My consulting room looked like a war zone. There were blood splashes on me, on Fiona, on the walls and on the floor. My computer keyboard was smothered in red dots, the couch was soaked and Josie's boots underneath it were fit only for the bin. None of that mattered, though. Lying peacefully in Josie's arms, the baby and her mother only had eyes for each other.

Because of the rapid delivery, Josie had torn badly, and the traumatised area around her vagina was bleeding profusely. We urgently needed to get her to hospital to have it sutured. Josie was also going to need expert help over the next few days to get used to the idea of being a mum and to be taught how to care for her little daughter.

I buzzed Doreen to say that the paramedics could come and take Josie now. Two of them came in carrying a stretcher which they almost dropped when they surveyed the carnage.

'You've had a busy morning,' commented one of them before helping his colleague to transfer Josie and her baby on to the stretcher.

I explained to Josie: 'You need to be in hospital for a bit, but it's nothing to be frightened about.'

'You did really well,' Fiona fibbed.

Just when I thought I could relax, and my mind drifted to thoughts of that long-delayed coffee, Josie hit me with another challenge as she was being wheeled out. 'Doctor, I don't have my mobile with me,' she said. 'Could you call my mum and let her know where I am? I think she would understand better if it came from you.'

I tried to wriggle out of it but Josie was adamant. 'She'll murder me – you've got to tell her,' she said.

I had a brief image of yet more blood. 'OK,' I said somewhat half-heartedly. 'Can you . . . ?' I began, turning to Fiona.

'Certainly not,' she said, a tad brusquely. 'This is your call – I wouldn't mind listening in, though. I know Josie's mum and she doesn't pull her punches.'

'Well a bit more abuse will just roll off me now,' I said.

Before I made the call I had my overdue coffee, possibly the best I'd ever tasted. Josie's mother, Maria, was also a patient at the surgery and I asked for her notes so I could assess what sort of person I'd be dealing with and what her reaction might be. I discovered that Maria was being treated for depression by Nazareen, one of my female colleagues, and I saw a way out. What better person to break the news than a familiar face? Her own doctor could tell her. Naz has a great sense of humour and energy for life that would leave most people exhausted. She has three children under six years old, yet somehow manages to carry out a demanding, full-time job, attend the gym regularly to maintain her superb figure, and yet unashamedly indulges in a little too much alcohol on her precious weekly nights out with the girls. 'Those nights keep me sane,' she says. 'They remind me of how exciting I used to be before I became a mother!'

Unfortunately, though, Naz was on holiday.

The practice staff were wonderful and refused to let me clear up my bloody consulting room. 'Go and get yourself cleaned up,' said Doreen. 'You and Fiona both need a change of clothes, a shower and a hair wash. You look like extras from a Hammer Horror film and you'll terrify your patients looking like that.'

She was right. At home I saw that my blonde hair had acquired some unusual red highlights and that my new, pale blue cashmere sweater – ironically worn for the first time that day – looked like road kill. Although the label said 'machine washable', the blood never did come out.

Feeling drained, I took my time eating some cold, left-over pasta I'd found in the fridge. Then I drove to the flat that Josie and her mother shared on a nearby council estate. There was no reply when I knocked. I tried phoning, too, but no one picked up. I sat on the tenement stairs, feeling crushingly tired and wondering what to do next. Perhaps Josie's mum didn't even know her daughter hadn't come home as planned but, on the other hand, perhaps she was going crazy with worry and was out looking for her.

Finally, I put a note through her door on headed notepaper, asking her to contact the surgery. I added that Josie had to go to hospital unexpectedly, but that she was doing well and that there was nothing to worry about. I didn't want to scare her.

When I didn't hear anything for a couple of hours, I hoped that the hospital or Josie herself had contacted Maria and that I was off the hook. No chance.

Mid-afternoon during surgery, I heard loud voices coming from reception.

'Where's my Josie? What's happened to her?' a woman was shrieking.

I couldn't leave my room straight away because I had a patient with me but all the time I was aware of the escalating hysteria emanating from reception and that the woman – and I had no doubt who she was – was demanding to see me RIGHT NOW.

As soon as my patient left, Maria stormed in. 'Where is she? What's happened to my Josie? I want the truth. Why won't anyone tell me what's been going on?'

Josie's mum was small, plump and badly dressed. Although I had seen from her notes that she was forty, she looked ten years older. Life had clearly not treated Maria well. I wasn't sure where to start. Blurt it out straight away or take or more gentle approach?

'Josie came in here this morning with bad tummy pains . . .' I began.

'Yes, she was moaning about it this morning,' said Maria. 'I told her she'd been eating too many chips. Her tummy was so huge she looked pregnant.'

Here was my cue. 'Maria, your daughter was pregnant.'

Silence. Her jaw dropped. Suddenly it hit her.

'Pregnant? She can't be. I'd have known.'

I waited and Maria continued, 'Hang on. You said she was pregnant. What's happened? Has she lost the baby?'

'No, Maria, she's had a baby girl, here in my room, this morning. The baby's fine, and so is Josie.'

Maria just sat, open mouthed, staring at the wall behind me. I broke the silence.

'Josie's in the post-natal ward at the hospital. She needed a few stitches.'

Still no response. I waited. I had to give her time to take in what I'd just said.

Maria began to sob. She fished a hankie from inside her jumper and wiped her eyes. 'Why didn't she tell me?' she said quietly. 'She must have known she was pregnant. She probably thought I'd be angry – well, she'd have been right.'

'Maria, she genuinely didn't know,' I said. 'It was as big a surprise to her as it is to you now.'

'But I should have guessed. All those chips. She's always had a good appetite but she's never eaten like that before. Will the baby be OK? All she's been eating is chips and chocolate.'

'The baby looked fine. I don't think the chip diet has done her any harm at all. Josie was scared about telling you, though, that's why I put the note through your door.'

'I didn't want her to end up like me,' said Maria, 'and she knew that. I was engaged when I discovered I was pregnant at the age of eighteen. My fiancé didn't hang around and my mum chucked me out. I didn't want that for Josie. She's a clever girl – she's got two A levels and was in her first term at college – now this.'

'You don't have to chuck her out,' I ventured.

'No,' said Maria, 'I don't.'

'Give Josie my best wishes, please,' I said as she left the room. 'Tell her I'm looking forward to seeing her and the baby again.'

I wondered if I ever would. After the trauma of the birth and all those names she'd called me, Josie might decide that she never wanted to see me again.

I had underrated her.

Several months later a young woman came into my consulting room with a baby in her arms. I'd only quickly scanned my list and didn't recognise her name at first. I certainly did not recognise her when I saw her. Josie had lost a vast amount of weight and both she and the baby, who'd been named Kylie, glowed with good health.

'I don't eat chips anymore,' Josie told me when I commented on her slimmer figure. 'I've gone back to college. I do bar work to help pay for my keep and for Kylie, and my mum is being marvellous looking after her. You wouldn't recognise mum either, Doctor Leonard. Now she has a granddaughter to care for she doesn't seem so depressed – she's even coming off her pills. Kylie's the best thing that has ever happened to us. Still, I don't want any more babies yet, so that's why I've come to see you. I need to get myself protected – maybe a coil or an implant? I don't have a boyfriend but I'd like one just in case.'

I was amazed she had remembered my little talk – but she could recall much more than that.

'I did listen to you, Dr Leonard,' she said as she left. 'I remember everything that happened that day. You and that nurse, Fiona, were wonderful – and I was foul to you both. I'm so sorry for calling you a cow.'

CHAPTER THREE

TAKING A DEEP BREATH

Goodness, I thought, as I lifted the hefty bundle of paper, that's a mighty big set of notes for a sixteen-year-old.

I checked the date of birth on the front envelope. Yes, he really was only sixteen. What on earth had been going on? I grabbed the box of notes, said bye to the receptionists and headed home.

It was just before 8pm and my male nanny Adrian had just finished getting my boys tucked up into bed. I'd been so lucky to find him, especially as male nannies were pretty rare. I wouldn't have minded having a female nanny, but as a single mother with two boys, I had wanted a bloke in the job if possible. Adrian had come to England from New Zealand to improve his photography skills and worked as a nanny to fund the trip.

Although he had not done much formal training, he had a wonderful way with Thomas and William. He was a good, kind disciplinarian and gained the respect of us all. Adrian and I had a flexible arrangement which seemed to work well for us both. He would work all the hours I wanted if he could get time off for his car photography, when he would travel to rallies and race tracks all over the country. Thomas, my oldest son, had been interested in cars ever since he was a toddler, and having Adrian around fuelled his passion, and today he's a real petrol head. Adrian was an excellent role model for the boys, in all sorts of ways, and very supportive of me. As well as taking care of my sons, he helped with the cooking, washing and ironing, so they have not grown up thinking that all the everyday boring household chores are solely the province of women and far too demeaning for a man to tackle.

I'd arrived home just as he was finishing their bedtime story, and had given them both a big hug and goodnight kiss. Must get home earlier tomorrow, I thought. My turn to do the story and spend some time with them.

I resisted the urge to pour myself a glass of wine and instead lit the fire in the front room and sat down on the sofa with my work. I began ploughing my way through a pile of notes that needed what we called 'summarising'. After a new patient registers at the practice, their notes eventually arrive from their previous surgery (a process that could take anything from one month to a year) and, every week, each doctor was handed a bundle to go through at home. Our job was to get a basic medical summary on to the front sheet that would give easily accessible information whenever the patient came into the surgery. The notes were stored in buff envelopes, named after Lloyd George, who first introduced National Insurance back in 1911. At a size of 7 by 5 inches , and expanding to a depth of 4 inches when required, the records were made up of a set of cards for handwritten notes, lined blue for women and red for men. Typed letters from the hospital were folded together at the back. Both sets were held separately by a treasury tag. Most patients only needed one envelope for their entire records, though older people, especially those with complex medical problems, often expanded into two. And it was easy to spot patients who had seen private specialists, as the thicker paper they used for their letters soon filled up the envelopes. For a sixteen-year-old to have three bulging envelopes, so full they were falling apart, and held together with an elastic band stretched to breaking point, was highly unusual.

It soon became clear that this lad, Josh, had been registered with at least eight different doctors since he'd been born and his notes were a complete mess. Far from a neat pile in chronological order, I found notes from his baby days mixed in with notes from the previous year.

I cleared the coffee table and started making heaps for each year of his life. In every one I soon had a letter from a hospital following an admission for an acute asthma attack. Some years there were several. And then there were the letters from paediatric asthma clinics, documenting how difficult it was to control Josh's 'brittle' asthma. But there were an equal number of letters from the same clinics just informing the GP that Josh had failed to turn up for his appointment.

I then started on the GP's notes. Handwritten on loads of red cards, at least they were mainly in the right order, but even to my eye, trained in deciphering doctors' appalling handwriting, most were completely unintelligible. But I could pick out lots of comments about 'advice to Mum again to use inhalers regularly', and even more 'DNAs' – doctors' shorthand for Did Not Attend. After some of these the card was blank and the writing on the next one was completely different. I guessed he hadn't turned up because he'd moved. A picture soon emerged of a lad with severe asthma, whose care had been hopelessly disjointed. No wonder he had been admitted into hospital as an emergency, with a severe asthma attack, so many times. I discovered he'd even had to be put on a ventilator a couple of times.

The following day, I had a word with Fiona, who ran the asthma clinic at the surgery.

'We've a new patient, a sixteen-year-old lad called Josh – lives in one of the flats on the estate opposite. He's got dreadful asthma, which is very badly controlled. But I think the main problem is he's never had any continuity of care. I was going to call him in for an appointment.

If I sort his inhalers out, can you see him afterwards to check he's using them properly and then arrange a follow-up appointment?'

'Sure – if he's sixteen then he's certainly old enough to take charge of his asthma. I wonder how much he's been taught about it?'

'From looking at his records, not a lot. He's nearly died a couple of times, but as soon as he's come out of hospital he seems to have moved, so no one's been able to check on his care afterwards.'

I asked Lizzy, one of the receptionists, to try and get in contact with him.

'Tell him it's not urgent – I don't want him scared, but that I need to do a routine asthma check.'

He didn't turn up for his first two appointments. That tells a story, I thought to myself. But it was third time lucky. Dressed in baggy jeans, ripped across the knee, a huge hoodie, his trainers had soles so thick he couldn't flex his feet, and the untied laces were clearly for decoration only. His look was completed by a baseball cap placed on his head, not only at an angle, but back to front. A young woman – who looked barely in her twenties, came with him.

'Hello doc, I hear you want to talk about my asthma. It's not a problem now, but mum here insisted I come.' Phew, good thing I didn't call her his girlfriend, I thought.

'He never thinks it's a problem, until he's admitted to the hospital unable to breathe,' she chipped in. 'That's why I made him come in. I can't keep reminding him to take his inhalers. Especially at his age.'

'Josh, which inhalers are you using at the moment?' I wondered if he knew.

'Just the blue one. The last doctor I saw gave me a brown one to use, but that didn't seem to do anything, so I stopped it.'

'How often did you use the brown one?' I asked.

'When my breathing was bad – just like the blue one. But, as I said, I don't use it now. It didn't help at all. It's only the blue one that helps.'

I realised immediately why Josh had been into hospital so many times. It was time to go back to basics. I explained that there were two main types of inhaler for treating asthma. 'Your blue inhaler is what we call a "reliever". It contains the drug salbutamol, which widens your airways. When you have an asthma attack your airways become narrowed and reliever inhalers help to widen them up again. The brown one the other doctor gave you is what's called a "preventer". As their name suggests, this type of inhaler helps to stop the airways becoming inflamed and narrowed in the first place. But they don't have any immediate benefit. For them to work they have to be used regularly, every day, even when you breathing feels OK.'

'Don't they help when my breathing's bad?'

'No, that's why you found that the brown one didn't seem to make any difference when you'd been wheezing.'

'So I need to use it all the time?'

'Yes. The aim of good asthma treatment is to stop those wheezing attacks. With good preventer treatment you should hardly ever have to use your blue inhaler.'

'Well, that's never going to happen. That's the one that works for me. As long as I use it all the time, I can breathe properly. You're not going to stop me using my blue inhaler.'

I could see educating Josh about his asthma was going to be a bit of an uphill struggle, but his mother at least was encouraging.

'C'mon, Josh, we don't want any more scares with you being rushed into hospital, unable to breathe and going blue. Listen to what the doctor's saying.'

There was one more thing I wanted to tackle.

'You've moved around an awful lot recently. Was there any particular reason for that? Are you likely to be around here for long?'

I wanted to know how long Fiona, I and the rest of the team at the surgery had to get Josh's asthma sorted out.

'I've had problems with my ex-partner. Not Josh's dad, his younger brother's dad. He kept beating me up and has threatened Josh as well, and I've had to take out an injunction against him to stop him coming near us. Had to keep moving to get away from him. But now he's behind bars for at least five years, so I'm hoping we can stay put here for a while, and Josh and his brother can settle into college.'

I was curious to know what on earth the man had done to be 'care of Her Majesty' for so long, but I thought that could wait. No doubt someone in the surgery would find out, sooner or later. But the story went some way to explaining why so many hospital appointments had been missed. I guessed the family had been moving at very short notice. Not only that, but clearly life for Josh had hardly been all peace and calm. I wondered how many of his attacks had been triggered by stress from a fight going on at home.

'Great. I'll give you a prescription for two of each type of inhaler, so even if you can't find one, you have a spare, but it's important you use them properly. Could you pop down and see nurse Fiona, and she'll make sure the medicine is going where it's needed, which is into your lungs. And then can you come back in a month, so we can see how you are getting on?'

I caught up with Fiona later in the day.

'He hadn't a clue how to use an inhaler,' she commented. 'Taking umpteen puffs and swallowing nearly all of it. I think he's got the hang of it now, though, and I've given him lots of leaflets to read – though of course whether he'll open them or not is another matter . . .'

He was back sooner than we had expected.

I was the duty doctor, it was the end of the afternoon, and I just finishing off dealing with a pile of repeat prescriptions, when my phone rang. It was Lizzy.

'That new lad, Josh, he's just come in, wheezing really badly. Think he needs seeing straight away.'

I hurried downstairs and could see – and hear – straight away that Josh, who was on his own, was having an acute asthma attack. I took him straight into one of the nurse's rooms, which was empty, and pulled out the nebuliser kit from the cupboard. A nebuliser is a device that turns a liquid form of medicine into a fine mist that can be breathed into the lungs. I emptied a small vial of salbutamol, the medicine that widens the airways, into a chamber attached to a mask, which I gently placed over Josh's face. The chamber was connected via plastic tubing to the machine.

'I'm sure you've used one of these before?' He nodded. 'Just breathe normally. And try to ignore the racket. One day someone will invent one of these machines that's a bit quieter. But first, could you take these?' I handed him ten steroid pills, a dose of 50mg, which would hopefully reduce some of the inflammation in his airways that was making them so narrow.

'What? All of them? Together?'

'Yes, though you can take them one by one if you prefer. It's either that or I'll have to give you an injection.'

'I'll take the pills. Somehow.' He managed a brief smile, while I filled up a plastic cup with some water.

Normally giving a patient with an acute asthma attack a dose of nebulised salbutamol rapidly improves their breathing, but I could see within a couple of minutes that it wasn't having much of an effect on Josh. I dashed into reception, where Lizzy was packing up.

'Could you get an ambulance for me please. As quickly as possible. Blue light. Josh's breathing is really bad and he needs to be in hospital.'

Asking for a 'blue light' ambulance means it's a real emergency, and coming from a doctor's surgery, I knew one would be on its way very fast. But it had to get through the 6pm rush hour traffic.

The first dose of salbutamol had finished, and Josh was still gasping, and using his chest muscles to try and get air into his lungs.

'I'll give you another dose while we wait. Don't worry; the ambulance will be here soon. Just take slow, deep breaths, try not to breathe too fast.'

The second dose was just coming to an end, with seemingly little effect on his breathing, as the ambulance arrived. They hooked him up to an oxygen cylinder and attached monitors for his pulse and the amount of oxygen in his blood stream – which was alarmingly low. It should have been at least ninety-eight per cent. Instead it was only ninety-two. It may not sound a big difference, but just that small drop could be life threatening.

'Don't worry, lad, we'll soon have you down at the hospital.' The older of the two male members of the crew had clearly seen many scenes like this before.

After they'd gone, I realised I ought to try and locate Josh's mother. There was no reply to the phone and, as it wasn't far, I popped over the road towards their flat. She was walking along the path as I arrived.

'Dr Leonard, hello,' she smiled at me. 'You're out a bit late. Is it one of the old folk in the block?'

'No, it's Josh. I've just sent him off in an ambulance to the hospital. Another asthma attack.'

'That stupid boy. I kept reminding him to use the new brown inhaler, but I don't think he did. Said it wasn't any good for his breathing.'

'When he comes out of hospital, will you get him to come and see me or Fiona again? Tell him we're not going to tell him off – we're there to help him. And to stop him having to go through another episode like this evening. And tell him I don't want to go grey, not just yet anyway.'

She grinned, 'You're not the only one.'

I was tired when I got home. The boys were eating tea at the kitchen table. I noticed that William was coughing occasionally.

'He's been doing that since he came home from school,' Adrian explained. 'But he's not ill, no temperature, and that's his second helping of apple pie. I don't think there's much wrong with him.'

William grinned at me from across the table.

'Can you help me with my Lego pirate ship when I've finished?'

As I was attaching the sail to the mast, I noticed he was still coughing, but didn't seem remotely troubled by it. It was early November and the season for coughs and colds was just starting. Not only that, but William, now aged six, had just switched schools and was being exposed to a new, larger set of boys and their germs. It was likely he would get at least one nasty cold or cough this winter. And as nearly all illnesses like that are caused by viruses, there was nothing I could do about it. I wasn't remotely concerned.

Josh was back in the surgery, a few days later, with his mother. He'd just completed a course of steroids and the hospital had switched him to a higher dose of 'preventer' inhaler.

'Josh, you've really got to use this one. I know you don't think it does any good but, please, give it a chance. Used regularly, it really will help to stop those nasty acute attacks.'

'But they're not dangerous.'

'Josh, asthma can be very dangerous. Three people die every day from asthma in the UK.'

'But not young people like me. You're talking about older people.'

'No, Josh, I'm talking about young people, just like you.'

'You're kidding me?'

'No, I'm not. I read recently that twenty-seven children aged less than fourteen died from asthma last year.'

'That's not many.'

'It's twenty-seven too many. Almost certainly none of them need have died if their asthma had been controlled properly.'

'OK, OK. So what do I need to do?'

Ideally I wanted him to keep a record of how often he used both his inhalers. That would give me a good idea of how well controlled his asthma was. The less he used his blue inhaler – his reliever – the better. But I needed to be realistic. Josh, keeping a record? I didn't think that was going to happen.

'Just try to remember to use that new brown inhaler, two puffs, twice a day. If you forget, use it as soon as you remember. I'd prefer you had too much rather than too little.'

'I don't want to nag you, Josh,' his mother added in, 'but all these dramas with your breathing are getting too much for me. And it's not fair on your brother either. Time you grew up a bit. You're nearly seventeen now.'

'OK, Mum, sorry. I'll try, honest I will.'

I had to dash off early that day to hear Thomas, who was learning the saxophone, play in a pupils' concert at school. Held at least three times a term, it was a way of getting boys used to playing in front of an audience; all ages, and standards, were represented. Some of the older boys were really accomplished musicians and I felt sorry for their parents, sitting listening to one of the smaller boys screeching out a rather tuneless 'Twinkle, twinkle, little star' on a pint–sized violin. I was grateful that neither of my two had chosen to learn a string instrument. Somehow listening to a beginner on a saxophone or clarinet – William's choice of instrument – wasn't too painful on the ears. William sat beside me – I knew he'd be performing in one of these concerts in the not-too-distant future, so it was good for him to experience what went on and to hear how well the older boys could play. But sitting in the quiet of the music room, William's cough was more noticeable – and disruptive. We left as soon as Thomas had played.

I checked with William whether he felt unwell, or breathless.

'No, mum, I'm fine. Just got a cough. And my nose is bunged up a bit now, as well,' he added, wiping the green goo coming out of his nostrils on the sleeve of his jumper.

'Any chance I could get you to use a tissue for that?'

He gave me another of his cheeky grins.

Back in the surgery, it was Fiona who updated me on Josh's progress.

'Wonders will never cease. He actually kept his appointment with me today. His inhaler technique has improved, but I'm really not sure how often he's using the preventer. His peak flow is still too low for my liking, so I've upped the dose. Hope that's OK.'

The peak flow is a measure of how fast someone can breathe out. It's a useful way of monitoring asthma – generally the lower the reading, the more narrow the airways, and vice versa.

'I've also given him a peak-flow monitor to use at home, and asked to him to write down the measurements, at least once a day.'

I raised my eyebrows.

'OK, I know there isn't a hope he'll do it that often,' she admitted, 'but just twice a week would be progress.'

But ten days later, midday Friday, Josh was back, with yet another acute attack. This time I could see from the moment that he walked in that he needed to go to hospital – fast. I asked Doreen, who was on the desk, to call a blue light ambulance straight away, then got Josh hooked up again to the nebuliser. His shoulders were going up and his ribs were moving heavily as he used every muscle he possessed to try and get air into his lungs. This time, I gave him an even larger dose of steroid, by injection, straight into one of his veins.

Yet again the emergency treatment I gave him in the surgery only improved his breathing very slightly. I was very grateful when, yet again, the ambulance turned up quickly. And, very unusually, it was the same crew.

'You're getting to be quite a regular, young lad. Let's get you into the back of the van and to hospital.'

I went up to the kitchen to get a cup of coffee and met Fiona and Naz.

'We're not doing very well here, are we? He's had two attacks within a month. He's on the maximum dose of preventer inhaler. Do you think we need to give him a longer course of steroids to take by mouth?'

'Are you sure he's actually using his inhalers?' Naz asked. 'Taking oral steroids when he's still growing should be pretty much last resort.'

It was Fiona who voiced what I was thinking. 'He just doesn't seem to be able to take his asthma seriously. Rosemary's told him, and so have I, that it can be fatal, but I honestly don't think he believes us.'

'Has he got an appointment booked at the asthma clinic at the hospital?' Naz asked. 'We need some expert help with him.'

'He had an appointment after his last emergency admission but, guess what? He didn't turn up.'

'And his mother was furious with him,' I added, 'which I understand, but I don't think it's helping the situation. I think things are really strained between them. She's working full-time and can't keep taking time off to go with him to appointments. And I think Josh's brother is a bit of a troublemaker, and it can't help that his father is in prison.'

I thought of my two young boys at home. I knew that adolescent boys could be a handful. I only hoped mine didn't cause me too much trouble.

As always, I was glad when the weekend came. Time to slow down, get some sleep, and do some sport with the boys. Only William still had a heavy cold, which meant that swimming was off the agenda. But, other than that, I didn't pay much attention to his health. Like most GPs I knew, I was exposed to so much illness in my working life that I tended to shrug off minor illness in my family. Both of them had hardly had a day off school, and probably sometimes thought of me, with justification, as a rather unsympathetic mother.

Taking a Deep Breath

On Sunday afternoon Thomas was out playing with a friend and William was quietly occupied playing in his room – or so I thought. I was repairing the tears in three pairs of school trousers when he came into the study, coughing worse than before, and visibly gasping for breath.

'Mum, I can't breathe.'

I was horrified. He was obviously having an asthma attack. I grabbed the spare stethoscope I kept in my desk drawer and had a listen to his chest. His lungs were wheezing badly. All over.

Unlike now, when doctors' visiting bags are kept at the surgery, I had my own visiting bag at home with an emergency supply of drugs. The salbutamol inhaler was buried at the bottom and I had to empty out nearly the whole contents of the bag to get to it.

I showed William what to do and, as he sat, breathless, he slowly took ten puffs, the large dose that is used when someone is wheezing badly. He stayed remarkably calm. It helped a bit, but it was clear his chest was still very tight. I didn't think he necessarily needed to be admitted to hospital but he needed to be nebulised. And not by me. Now was the time for me to be a mother, not a doctor. I rang the out of hours' service, and arranged for the duty doctor to see William straight away.

Thankfully I knew Dick, the duty doctor, very well. He was a senior colleague at a neighbouring practice.

As William sat breathing the vapour of salbutamol

through the nebuliser mask, I answered the questions I knew were coming.

'So, how long has he had a cough?'

'I'm not sure. Probably about a month.'

'And you never suspected it was asthma?'

'No. I just assumed it was a viral cough. He was never ill or short of breath – until today.'

'Was the cough worse after he did any exercise, or at night.'

'I don't know. I didn't notice . . .'

I felt mortified that I could have been so negligent about my own son's health. But Dick was reassuring.

'We've all done it, Rosemary. Everyone knows that medical parents fall into two categories. There are the ones that worry about every little thing, and have their kids in and out of doctors' surgeries the whole time and on medicines they probably don't need. And then there are the ones like you – and me, I might add – who tend to ignore their kids, healthwise. If it makes you feel any better, I heard last week about a medical colleague whose kid had been complaining about a painful ankle for a couple of weeks. His doctor dad just told him he'd twisted it and to stop moaning. It was his mum who finally took him to get the X-ray that showed two broken bones.'

The nebuliser treatment worked well for William but his asthma attack was severe enough to warrant treatment with a course of steroids, by mouth. He was also started on a preventer inhaler, and I had a very similar conversation with him to the one I'd had with Josh a few weeks previously.

'So, if I use this brown one every day, I won't cough or get breathless?'

'Yes, that's the idea.'

'Well, that's easy. It was horrible not being able to breathe. Don't want that happening again.'

I gave him a big hug and we agreed that even though he was only six, I would leave him in charge of his inhalers, though Adrian or I would check that he hadn't forgotten.

'But don't worry if you do,' I added; 'everyone forgets now and again.'

'I'm not going to,' he said proudly.

He turned out to be as human as everyone else, but the times he forgot were few and far between. And very soon we discovered the thing that triggered his asthma – having a cold. We learnt that as soon as his jumper sleeve started being used as a nose wipe, it was time to increase his dose of preventer inhaler.

Josh was kept in hospital for a week after his latest attack and his treatment regime was altered again. Montelukast, a treatment taken by mouth, was added into the mix, along with a yet more powerful preventer.

He came in to see me a couple of weeks later.

'Have to tell you, Dr R, that you and Fiona here are a lot nicer than the doctors and nurses at the hospital. They gave me a right talking to. Told me off, which I didn't like. Treated me like I was five. I'm not going back to see them again.'

That's because you act like a five-year-old, I thought silently. Particularly when it comes to your asthma. If my six-year-old can use his inhaler regularly...

'But what about your out-patient appointment?'

'Forget it, I'm not going to be spoken to like that. I can get my check-ups and medicines from you, can't I?'

'Of course, but promise me, please, that you'll use your inhalers properly and take the pills regularly.'

'OK, then.'

Interesting, I thought. Teenagers are tricky. The hospital doctors got cross with him and, on the one hand, it seems to have got the message home that he needs to take his medicine or he's going to end up having to face them again as an in-patient. But he won't go back to see them for a clinic appointment.

Josh only came up on my radar again at a practice meeting five months later.

'Anyone heard anything from Josh?' asked Fiona, as we were going through the list of patients who had been causing us some concern. 'Only he hasn't turned up for his last two asthma clinic appointments. Have the family moved again?'

I went and collected his records. They were easy to find, as he was now on to envelope number four. All I had to do was look for the biggest bundle in the drawer.

'As far as I can tell he's still with us.'

'Has he been ordering his inhalers?'

I had a look at his cards and, from what I could see, he hadn't asked for any medicines for three months, which was worrying. But we agreed that it was not our job to check up on a seventeen-year-old. And, after all, lots of patients fail to turn up for appointments – we couldn't try and contact all of them. We simply didn't have time.

The following Monday, I'd just got up to my room, when Doreen buzzed through to me.

'Rosemary, can you come down to reception? There's a fax I think you need to see.'

This was unusual. Usually the faxes – a big pile of them, reporting on the treatment our patients have received from the out-of-hours service, are just put in the duty doctor's box.

I went downstairs to see both Doreen and Lizzy visibly shaken and upset.

They silently put the printed sheet in front of me.

'I regret to inform you,' it began, 'that Josh Taylor, date of birth 10.5.80, died in this hospital on . . .'

It gave Saturday evening's date and then told me a full summary would follow.

No. Surely not? I was stunned.

Doreen broke the silence, 'I'll phone A&E and find out what happened.'

It was difficult to get going on my normal work but, as usual on a Monday morning, my surgery was packed.

Doreen came in, half-way through, with a mug of coffee.

'It was asthma. Being a Saturday, we weren't open. He went to A&E and they tried everything. But they couldn't save him.' Tears were welling up in her eyes.

'Has anyone heard anything from his mother?'

'No, but I'll drop her a note – a bit more than the usual condolence letter, though. She's going to need your care now.'

It was actually Fiona, the practice nurse, who was able to piece the story together – from both Josh's mother and his younger brother. After his last admission, Josh had initially been very good about using his medication. He had taken his tablets and used his preventer inhalers regularly. And his breathing had been fine. Back to normal, his brother had said. And the more normal he felt, the less he had bothered to use his inhalers. And then he hadn't bothered to take his tablets. And then, over a period of a few days, he had become short of breath. He'd started his inhalers again, but then his breathing had become worse and it was too late.

Could any of us have done any more? Should I have been tougher with him? Spelt out the dangers more clearly?

I just don't know.

CHAPTER FOUR

BEATING THE ODDS

I became a doctor because I wanted to save lives and ease suffering. There's a big downside to the job, though, and you need to be extremely tough to cope with it.

Even after more than twenty years as a GP, seeing a nasty result that could mean a patient has a terminal illness always brings a lump to my throat. I always dread breaking bad news. I may have had lots of training on how to do it, but that doesn't make it any easier.

Telling someone that they have run out of options, and that they are going to die in the near future is dreadful. Yet it's something I've had to do ever since I qualified and, like all doctors, I have to remain professional because it wouldn't help the patient to see their GP nearly breaking down in tears. I wait until I get home to do that.

Doctors may know a lot about the human body but we don't know it all, especially when it comes to the power of the mind and its ability to conquer overwhelming physical odds. So there's always hope and just occasionally there are wonderful surprises.

I'd known Gordon from almost the first week I'd started work as a GP in south London. Like all the male members of his family, he had high blood pressure and, despite a healthy lifestyle, he'd been on medication since his mid-forties.

Gordon was always immaculately turned out when he came to see me. Now that he had retired from his work, he had swapped his city suits for a more casual look – sports jacket, cords, a flannel shirt and his old Cambridge college tie – but he hadn't let his standards drop. I could almost have used his highly polished brown brogues as a mirror. Initially, I'd thought he must have spent some time in the Army, but he denied this – he just said he had been brought up to take pride in his appearance and that polishing your shoes only took a few minutes if you did it regularly.

I liked Gordon immensely and that had nothing to do with his dapper appearance. What endeared him to me most was his positive view of life and his sunny disposition. He always came into my consulting room with a smile and, even on the rare occasions when he was ill, as opposed to having a routine check-up, he never complained.

As I called him into my room on this particular day, I noticed that he was bearing a large takeaway cup from the café next door.

'I reckon you could do with this,' he told me. 'You're obviously having one hell of a morning and I bet that one is cold,' he added, pointing to the half-empty mug on my desk and handing me the steaming cup.

He was right. I'm a bad time-keeper, but that day I was running much later than usual and Gordon had waited an hour to see me. I marvelled that the new cup of coffee was piping hot – he'd obviously been keeping track of when he was going to be seen and had organised the coffee from the café next door to be ready at the right time.

'Sorry, and thank you. Yes, it's not been easy today,' I admitted. 'How are you, though? How's your blood pressure?' I knew that he kept track of it himself at home.

'It's OK,' Gordon replied. 'I'm not here about that – it's my lower back. It's been giving me a bit of gyp for several months and it's stopping me doing things I want to do, like digging the garden. I've had some physiotherapy but it hasn't really helped. The physio suggested that I come and see you.'

'That's sensible of her,' I replied. I asked when the pain had started and if Gordon could link its onset to anything unusual he'd been doing at the time.

'I can't think of anything,' said Gordon. 'No new physical exercise. I've been doing the garden, but I've been doing that for years. And I've not had an injury that might have triggered it.'

He added that the pain had come on very gradually and that the discomfort was limited to his back. He didn't have any pain down his legs, which can indicate pressure on the sciatic nerve.

When I examined Gordon I discovered that he had a tender area in the upper part of his lower back. It was in a slightly unusual place – most lower back problems occur further down, just above the buttocks, but even so I thought the most likely cause was 'wear and tear'. That's the euphemism for osteoarthritis, where the cartilage that protects the surface of bones within joints becomes worn. In his case, I suspected this had happened in one or two of the joints between the vertebrae, the individual bones of his lower spine.

As the pain was in a slightly odd place, however, and because physiotherapy had not alleviated it, I arranged for Gordon to have an X-ray.

'We need to check if there are any abnormalities in the bones. I'm not expecting to find any, though, other than maybe a touch of arthritis, but we need to be sure.'

When the result arrived in my in-tray a few days later, I received a nasty shock. Instead of the X-ray showing the slight changes to be expected in a man of sixty-seven, the report suggested that the first of the big lumbar vertebrae (L1) had collapsed.

No wonder Gordon had back problems – the collapsed bone itself could cause agonising pain, and the change in the structure of his spine would cause spasms in the surrounding muscles, which would only add to it.

The most common reason for the collapse of a vertebra is osteoporosis, which causes the bones to become so thin and fragile that they simply crush under the weight of those above them. It used to be common in women over seventy-five and is responsible for the classic curve of the upper back seen in some old women – the so-called 'dowager's hump'. Thankfully, with increasing awareness and preventative measures, such as taking extra calcium and medicines to help maintain bone structure, it is now becoming far more rare.

Although X-rays cannot be used to diagnose osteoporosis accurately – that can only be done with a special DEXA scan – they can reveal thinning of the bones. Osteoporosis doesn't occur in just one bone of the spine – it tends to happen to the whole lot. So when one collapses for this reason, the rest usually look pretty ropey, too. However, Gordon's X-ray results didn't conform to this type. The rest of his spine looked OK. He had just that one collapsed vertebra. I realised straight away that, in someone of his age, at the top of the list for possible causes for this problem was cancer.

I had a lump in my stomach as I looked at the results, willing them to show something different. My phone call to him was not something I could do in a rush, so I waited until I had a spare half-an-hour a little later in the morning. As always, I had a dilemma about how much to tell the patient. I wasn't sure Gordon had cancer – far from it.

That diagnosis could only be made after the bone had been biopsied, and I didn't want to scare him. After all, it was possible he had some rare form of osteoporosis that had affected just one bone.

The phone was answered by his wife Sheila.

'I've sent him out to Sainsbury's. He's been getting anxious about his back, so I decided to keep him occupied,' she cheerfully explained. 'He's always making comments about the cost of the weekly shop, so I thought he could do it himself to see where the money goes.'

I didn't want to worry Sheila, so I just asked her to get Gordon to phone me when he got home.

Half-an-hour later I took his call.

'Hello Doctor Leonard, it's Gordon phoning back as you requested. How are you?'

It was typical of him to ask after me when I knew he was so worried himself.

'I'm fine,' I said, 'but I wanted to discuss your X-ray report. It's a bit odd. Not what I was expecting.'

'I would ask if it's better or worse but, since you've rung me so quickly, it has to be the latter,' he replied.

I explained that one of his vertebrae had collapsed and that we needed to find out why. I asked him to come into the surgery so I could do a thorough physical examination and organise some blood tests.

'Could this be very bad news?' asked Gordon. 'Be honest, doctor, please.'

I took a deep breath. He'd asked me to be honest, so I

was. 'This type of problem is usually due to osteoporosis, Gordon, but the rest of your vertebrae look OK, so that means we do need to be sure it isn't something more serious.'

'Like cancer?'

'Yes,' I said. There was a horrible silence at the other end of the line.

Then he continued bravely, 'Under the circumstances, my wife might forgive me for forgetting to buy any milk or washing powder at the supermarket. When do you want to see me and should I bring her along, too?'

How typical of Gordon to make light of the situation and to spare me by being so pragmatic and sensible.

I booked him into one of the afternoon slots reserved for urgent patients. Normally these are opened up for booking only after 2pm and we use them for real emergencies. I didn't think my practice manager – who had to police the system – would complain in this case.

I called Gordon and Sheila into my room. Sometimes it can be daunting when a GP discovers that a patient has brought along a friend or a relative for moral support, especially if you suspect that they are not happy with the treatment they have received. A doctor can feel very threatened and very much on the back foot. Sometimes this tactic is used by patients to pressurise their doctor. On one occasion a patient brought a rather large friend along to try to make me refer him, unnecessarily in my opinion, to a specialist. When I refused and his friend started shouting and thumping the table to try to get his way, Doreen miraculously appeared.

'You don't speak to the doctor like that,' she told the two men, giving them the sort of look that would freeze vodka and was no doubt the same voice she used to keep her sons in line. 'Please leave now.'

Doreen is what author Alexander McCall Smith would call a traditionally built woman (in other words, large) with an enormous bosom in which beats a big but extremely cynical heart. I'd guess that she's an H-cup, though I'd never dare ask.

Although she was born in Britain, Doreen's parents came from the West Indies in the fifties and her dad found work on the London Underground. The oldest of eight children, it was Doreen who brought up her siblings, while her mum worked as a machinist, and it was she who took them to the doctors after grilling them mercilessly to make sure they were genuinely ill. This makes her brilliantly qualified for the job she does now. Doreen has no time for malingerers, which makes her unpopular with some of our patients. However, we'd be lost and completely overwhelmed without her sorting out the wheat from the chaff.

'How did you know I needed help?' I asked when they had left.

'I heard them talking strategy in the waiting room,' she said. 'The friend's a bit notorious around here. I've heard he's a regular in the local court and he's done time. He's a nasty bit of work and I wasn't going to leave you alone with that pair for very long.'

In Gordon's case, though, seeing him and Sheila together made sense – they could both hear the news delivered by the same person in the same way. It meant one of them did not have to rely on reported speech, which can sometimes be as bad as playing Chinese whispers. I've had numerous phone calls from worried partners who have had information relayed to them incorrectly. Seeing this couple together also meant there was a second person to ask questions which might not have occurred to the patient.

I'd met Sheila a few times before and, as always, she was as immaculately turned out as her husband, wearing a smart, navy blue, linen suit and white blouse. Her blonde hair was glossy and beautifully styled and she wore just the right amount of make-up to enhance her looks. She was ten years younger than Gordon and in her early fifties.

I showed them both the X-ray report and they held it between them while they read it through.

'Is it possible to see the actual films?' Sheila asked very reasonably. It was something patients often requested

'I wish,' I replied. 'I'd love to be able to see them myself. But no, they're kept at the hospital. You should be able to see them when you go there, though.'

'It mentions here possible metastases,' said Gordon after studying it carefully. 'That means there could be a cancer somewhere else in my body.'

I nodded. 'Yes, metastases are deposits of cancer cells in a different part of the body from the original site. They are sometimes called "secondaries". It's a sign that cancer has spread. They've mentioned metastases because it would be very unusual to get a primary cancer in one of the bones of the back – cancer in them is nearly always a secondary from somewhere else.'

'But where could the main cancer site be?' he continued. 'I seem completely well. In fact, since I retired and have had more time to exercise and take care of myself, I feel better than I have done for years.'

My first thought, given Gordon's age, was that he may have a prostate problem, especially as prostate cancer commonly spreads to bones. But he told me he had no problem with urine flow and never needed to get up to go to the loo during the night, which are the usual symptoms. 'I reckon I'm lucky there,' he commented. 'Most of my friends seem to be having problems in that department.'

I asked some general questions about Gordon's health – any weight loss, tiredness, loss of energy?

'No – I feel very fit,' he said. 'I've still got a healthy appetite – I can eat anything – I never have any stomach problems and I use the loo at the same time every morning.'

'Gordon!' remonstrated his wife.

'That's fine,' I laughed. 'I was going to ask.'

There was absolutely nothing in Gordon's history to give any clue where the primary cancer might be. And a physical examination proved similarly unhelpful. Gordon genuinely seemed perfectly well and even his back was more mobile and less sore than before.

I organised blood tests to check for anaemia, liver or kidney abnormalities and a stool test to check for hidden (occult) blood. Blood in the faeces can be a sign of something fairly minor, like piles, but it can also be a sign of inflammation in the lining of the intestine, or of cancer. And though sometimes it is obvious to see, as red streaks on the outside of the motions, or on toilet paper when you wipe yourself, sometimes the stools can look completely normal, but contain tiny amounts of blood, which can only be detected in the laboratory.

The whole lot came back absolutely normal. Neither I, nor he, were any the wiser and I was beginning to wonder whether the X-ray report had been wrong.

The next step was to refer Gordon to a bone specialist at the hospital, who arranged a more detailed computerised X-ray, called a CT scan, of Gordon's spine and abdomen. This confirmed that there was indeed something very wrong with his L1 vertebra. But otherwise it was completely normal.

A sample of tissue was taken from the abnormal bone and, sadly, this confirmed the original X-ray report findings. There were adenocarcinoma cells present – cancer cells originating from glandular tissue.

But glandular tissue from where? Where was the 'primary' site? Glandular tissue is found not only in the glands that produce hormones, such as the thyroid or the adrenals, but also in numerous other places, such as the kidneys and the whole of the gastro-intestinal tract, from the mouth to the anus. It could be anywhere in his body. Could the fact that he had no symptoms indicate that the culprit was the pancreas? Pancreatic cancer is notorious for being 'silent', and not causing any symptoms until it is at an advanced stage. However, if his pancreas was abnormal that should have shown up on the CT scan. It was a complete puzzle.

Gordon's digestive tract was then examined using tiny cameras, or endoscopes. His bowel was clear but a gastro-scopy, which examined the upper part, revealed a small red lump at the lower end of his oesophagus, the pipe that takes food from the mouth to the stomach. The specialist took a biopsy and, when the results came back two days later, they revealed that Gordon had cancer of the oesophagus.

I was dismayed but I was also very surprised. Normally cancer of the oesophagus causes discomfort behind the breast bone when eating a meal, and sometimes a sensation that food is getting stuck, especially if it isn't chewed into small pieces. But Gordon had no symptoms at all. Sheila even commented that, if anything, Gordon gobbled his meals and ate too fast.

When the couple came in to discuss the results with me, I didn't need to tell them how bad the diagnosis was – they had done their homework and had looked up cancer of the oesophagus on reputable websites.

'Because the cancer has spread to my bones, that indicates it's really advanced, doesn't it? Stage four, I think I read,' said Gordon. 'That means I need to get my affairs in order.'

Sheila was looking down and I knew she was trying hard not to cry. I wish I could have contradicted Gordon but he was right – the statistics for cancer of the oesophagus are indeed very depressing. Only thirty per cent of patients are alive one year after diagnosis, and just eight in one hundred survive for five years; and they are the ones who have caught the disease early. The outlook for Gordon, with an advanced stage four disease, was very grim.

Gordon decided to go ahead with a course of chemotherapy but he was realistic enough to know that it wasn't going to be a cure. 'It's just buying me a bit more time,' he said. 'If I feel really awful, I'll probably stop it. I want to be able to enjoy my last few months of life.'

'Absolutely,' I confirmed. 'Your choice. The cancer specialist and I will go along with whatever you want to do.'

'Something a bit more trivial, doctor, but important in its way,' he said. 'Before all this began with my back I booked a family holiday in Switzerland to celebrate Christmas and my birthday. My two children and four grandchildren are coming with us. It might be my last chance to have all the family round me but now I wonder if I will still be able to go?'

I could only tell him 'probably'. 'Why not wait until nearer the time before you make the final decision,' I said. 'You may not feel up to it.'

As expected, the course of chemotherapy took its toll on Gordon. Chemotherapy attacks all the rapidly dividing cells, which means not just cancer cells, but others such as those in the lining of the gut and the hair follicles. Gordon lost his hair, felt very sick and had bouts of diarrhoea, but he remained his usual cheerful self. He even managed to make jokes that for the first time in his long married life Sheila was encouraging him to eat more.

One of biggest problems for patients having chemotherapy is that the drugs also stop the production of white blood cells, which are an essential part of the body's immune system. This can make someone much more susceptible to infections than normal and a simple cold can easily turn into a nasty bout of pneumonia.

Four months into his course, Gordon's white cell count fell so perilously low that his next lot of treatment was delayed until the count had recovered a little. This meant the chemotherapy continued longer than expected and he had only just had his last injection when it was time to make the decision about whether he could go to Switzerland.

Gordon's white cell count was still low and I was concerned that sitting on a plane full of people, some of whom were bound to have coughs and colds, might not be in his best interests.

But he was adamant that he wanted to go. 'Come on, doctor, you know as well as I do that I may not get another chance for a trip like this. I know the family could all come and see me here in London but my grandchildren are looking forward to having some fun in the snow – and, actually, so am I.'

I tried to think as positively as he did. He wasn't going to the back of beyond and the healthcare in Switzerland is fantastic. So I gave him my blessing but advised him to check his holiday insurance policy very carefully. I didn't want him being landed with a huge bill if his condition worsened while he was away.

As he walked out of the door of my surgery I did have a thought that it might be the last time I saw Gordon. He looked so pale, thin and fragile and, for the first time, utterly beaten.

It was in the third week in January when I saw that Gordon was booked in to come and see me. I was really pleased to know he had made it back from his precious holiday seemingly without a medical crisis.

His appearance came as a complete and wonderful shock. The thin, frail man who had left the surgery before Christmas was gone. What a difference a month had made. Here was a slightly tanned, fit-looking man with a spring in his stride – the old Gordon was back.

'You look remarkably well.' I don't think I was able to keep the surprise out of my voice.

'Now I know why they have all those spas out there,' he

said. 'That fresh mountain air has done me a world of good. I even managed to do some skiing – I figured it was now or never.'

Gordon's blood tests showed his white cell count had recovered, too, but I wondered how long it would last. Although I said nothing, I knew he was thinking the same.

I kept expecting him to come back and tell me his back pain was worse or that he was having difficulty swallowing – signs that the cancer cells were growing again.

He saw his oncology specialist for regular check-ups every three months and after the third visit he came back to see me.

'Do I really need to keep going for check-ups like this?' he asked. 'I think I'm just wasting everyone's time – and, to be honest, it just reminds me that I ought to be ill by now. But I'm not, doctor, I feel fine. Could I just come to see you if I feel a twinge or something – then you'll be able to tell me if I need to go back to the hospital?'

So that's what we agreed to do.

I saw him next a couple of years later but interestingly both he and Sheila had booked appointments. They came in together.

'I thought I'd just report how well I'm feeling,' he said. 'Even my back pain has gone. So now it's Sheila's turn for some attention. I've dragged her along against her will – she's told me not to fuss, but she has really bad shoulder pain and I think it should be looked at.

'I reckon she's been suffering much more than me. We both know my time should be up by now – and that she's the one who is going to be left behind. She's been living on a knife edge and, to add to it all, she can't use her left arm properly.'

It emerged that for the past year Sheila, a left-hander, had been unable to move her left shoulder properly. She admitted that she'd had real difficulty changing gear while driving but had decided not to say anything because she thought it was minor compared with Gordon's problems.

She had a classic frozen shoulder. As its name suggests, movements of the shoulder are restricted and painful due to scar-like tissue forming round the joint. The condition usually starts out of the blue and is particularly common in women of Sheila's age.

She needed some physiotherapy and I was able to persuade her that Gordon could do without her for an hour a week while she took it. After all, he really did seem to be perfectly well.

Sheila popped in to see me at the end of her course of physiotherapy but sadly her shoulder wasn't much better. I needed to refer her to one of my colleagues for a steroid injection and, for the first time, she opened up about what she had been through.

'It's been surreal,' she told me. 'I've just been waiting for Gordon to die. Every time we do something together, I think, "this could be the last time". Even something simple, such as going out to lunch, has taken on ridiculous importance. And the weird thing is, I keep thinking to myself that I must enjoy each experience so that it becomes a happy memory, but I just can't.

'I've got to stop this now – I need to put Gordon's illness to the back of my mind. I'm even wondering if they made a mistake with the diagnosis. After all, how can he still be so well with stage four oesophageal cancer?'

She voiced what I had been thinking – had there been a mistake?

After she left I checked through all the notes, the X-rays and the biopsy reports. It was all there in black and white. There were cancer cells in the bone biopsy, a small picture of the red lesion in his oesophagus, and the biopsy report from the sample that was taken from it. A mistake about the diagnosis seemed very unlikely.

So what was the explanation? It is possible that the tumour had been there for years and was growing incredibly slowly. Perhaps the chemotherapy had killed it off? Either way, Gordon was beating all the odds.

I saw Gordon a few times over the following years and every time I saw his name on my list I felt an inward pang of nervousness. Had the cancer symptoms returned?

Eight years after his original diagnosis, his name was on my list again.

'Something new this time, doctor. I've had a trouble-some cough and vague chest discomfort for a couple of weeks. I got some cough medicine from the chemist, but it hasn't helped. I wonder if I've got a chest infection?'

Most likely that was exactly what he'd got and with any other patient I'd have either waited for it to get better, or have prescribed antibiotics. But with Gordon there was always the thought in my mind that the cancer had started growing again. I arranged for him to have a chest X-ray.

It was normal. No sign of an infection, or cancer, either. But ten days later he was back.

'Sorry to be a nuisance but the antibiotics haven't worked and, if anything, this discomfort in my chest is worse, especially when I try and do any exercise – I can't dig the garden and, though Sheila's shoulder is much better, I don't want her trying to do it instead of me.'

'Where exactly is the discomfort in your chest?' I asked him.

'It's a bit vague – sort of here,' he pointed, rubbing his chest on the left side. 'And it's not exactly pain. More of a pressure feeling.'

Another set of alarm bells rang. He was giving a very good description of angina, the discomfort that occurs when the heart muscle is deprived of oxygen. It's caused by a narrowing of one or more of the coronary arteries that supply blood to the heart.

'Gordon, I think it could be your heart,' I explained. 'We need to get you checked out at the hospital as soon as possible.'

I referred him to the Rapid Access Chest Pain Clinic – a relatively new system where patients with suspected heart problems are seen without delay.

The next thing I heard was from Sheila. 'I thought I'd phone and say thank you. One of his big coronary arteries was ninety per cent blocked. They've put in one of those metal coil things. He's making a good recovery. He'll be home in a couple of days.'

As usual, I'd heard nothing from the hospital. I was glad Sheila had let me know.

'It seemed that I was a heart attack waiting to happen,' Gordon admitted when he next saw me. 'Maybe I should have complained more about the pain but it honestly didn't seem that bad. And after all I'd been through . . .'

I wondered if Gordon had been mentally blocking out the pain, subconsciously fearing the cancer had returned and so he didn't want to know.

There's no doubt that having a stent – the 'metal coil thing' Sheila had described – inserted into one of the coronary arteries is a major medical procedure and, although most patients are out of hospital in a day or so, it can take several weeks to make a full recovery. So I wasn't that surprised when Sheila called me just under a month later.

'I just want to touch base with you,' she said. 'I'm worried about Gordon.'

Now I was worried, too – that was the first time I'd ever heard her say that. She continued: 'We've had friends who have had stents inserted because of angina and they've got better pretty quickly. But Gordon still looks pale and he is so tired. He's got absolutely no energy at all – he just wants to sit and do nothing – that's not like him at all.'

I offered to go round and see Gordon at home but Sheila refused, 'Oh no, I don't want to make work for you. He doesn't want to bother you, but I'll tell him I've already made an appointment so that he can't duck out of it.'

When they arrived, I could see immediately why Sheila was concerned. Gordon was pale and had lost weight again. Just walking to my consulting room had worn him out and he slumped into the chair by my desk.

'I'm just so weary,' he admitted. 'Even getting out of bed is an effort. I feel as bad as I did when I had the chemo. Whatever's been done to my heart, it hasn't helped at all. My chest still feels uncomfortable, too – is that usual?'

I knew it wasn't and once again I feared the worst. Had Gordon been fitted with a stent for nothing because the cancer had returned?

I arranged blood tests and an urgent chest X-ray and asked the hospital to fax me the result as soon as possible. I asked Doreen to buzz me as soon as it arrived.

The hospital was amazingly efficient and just three hours later the phone rang. 'Gordon's chest X-ray result is here,' said Doreen, 'and everything is OK.' She sounded as relieved as I felt. Like me, Gordon was one of her favourites. Doreen very much approved of people who, although they were really ill, never made a fuss.

Yet again, Gordon had given us another mystery to solve. What was causing his pain? I rang his oncologist and explained my concerns. I was convinced there was something serious going on but that I just hadn't found out where.

The oncologist arranged an immediate CT scan – a very detailed special type of X-ray – of Gordon's chest. It threw up a major surprise.

'He's got a large clot in one of the main veins inside his right lung – he's had a massive pulmonary embolus. By rights it should have killed him. It's amazing he's still alive,' he told me. That's occurred to me before, I thought to myself.

There was no way of knowing how long the clot had been there and I wondered whether it had been causing his chest pain all along. But if it had been found earlier, the coronary artery in his heart that apparently was about to block might never have been discovered. However you looked at it, Gordon was an incredibly lucky man.

He was treated with anti-coagulant drugs – first by injection, then daily tablets of warfarin, to thin the blood and prevent further clotting. Gradually Gordon's energy – and appetite – returned and three months later he was back to his usual energetic, happy self.

I saw him only last week and, rather unusually, he asked about my two pet cats.

'Why do you ask?'

'Well, they have nine lives and I wonder if I do, too. I've had three close scrapes, so that leaves me with another six.'

Beating the Odds

I didn't doubt it. I thought back to the day Gordon first came in with back pain. That was eight years ago. If someone had told me then that he would still be alive today, I just would not have believed it. All my training had taught me to be a non-sentimental realistic but it is really heartwarming when someone beats the odds. It's impossible to know when it's going to happen but Gordon is living proof that, no matter how dismal the prognosis, it is folly to give up on life – however many we think we have. And it also helps to have a partner who looks out for us, too.

CHAPTER FIVE

A HIDDEN AGENDA

'What do you mean, I don't need antibiotics? Of course I need them. My previous doctor always gave them to me when I had a cold.'

This was one of those days when I wished I was less conscientious. How wonderful it would have been to stay in bed, to pull the duvet over my head, just cop out, say that I was ill (which I seldom am) and avoid confrontations like this with unpleasant, unreasonable people.

It had been a fraught morning ever since I had reluctantly woken up with a sore throat and raspy voice. My oldest son Thomas had come into my bedroom mumbling that he did not feel well either. Having a mother like me, neither of my sons cries wolf, so I took him seriously. When I gave Tom a quick once-over I discovered he had a temperature and that the back of his throat was red. So now he was off school and I felt guilty about leaving him to go to the surgery. But I didn't feel ill enough to go off sick myself.

At times like that, when a child is ill, guilt sits on the shoulder of every working mum, and I was no exception. There were times when I felt that I was making a hash of both work and motherhood because I just couldn't wholeheartedly embrace either role. But like so many other mothers, I just muddled through, tried to do my best, and was, I hope, what I call 'a good-enough mother'.

However, I knew Thomas would be fine on a diet of paracetamol and TLC from Adrian, our nanny, but I still fretted. I had hoped for an early lunch break so I could dash home and reassure myself. The receptionists, aware that I was below par, had not added any extra patients to my surgery, and everything had been going to plan until this rude and angry man strode into my consulting room spoiling for a fight. Now I was in a stand-off situation and I had no intention of backing down. He had picked the wrong person and the wrong day. I was in zero tolerance mode for hypochondriacs. And, like every doctor I know, I don't like being treated like a secretary. I didn't go through six years of medical school just to write prescriptions without using some of my own judgement first.

Bob was over six feet tall, balding, overbearing, over-weight and trying to bully me. Perhaps he thought that size mattered but, although I'm only five feet two inches tall, I am not easily cowed. However, I was finding it hard to keep a pleasant look on my face during his rant. He had fleshy features and a pot belly spilled unattractively from his obviously expensive Savile Row suit. He wasn't doing his blood pressure any favours by getting so worked up, and mine was probably suffering, too. He struck the desk with his meaty fist and glared at me. Used to getting his own way, no doubt, both in the boardroom and at home, he had clearly planned to pop into the surgery, grab some drugs and then head to the office. My refusal to give in to his request had infuriated him.

'Colds are caused by viruses,' I said, wishing I had a pre-recorded tape to play every time I had to explain this to people, 'and antibiotics don't make any difference to viruses. They only deal with infections that are caused by bacteria.'

'But how do you know it's a virus and not bacteria?' he fumed. 'I've got all this green stuff coming from my nose. That means it's a bacterial infection, doesn't it? If it was just a virus it wouldn't be this revolting colour. You doctors think you know it all, but I know my own body and I need antibiotics.' Just to ram home his point, he thrust a hand into his suit pocket and I watched horrified as it emerged with a snot-covered handkerchief which he waved in front of my face. Great. I hoped I was already immune to what-ever bug was clearly flourishing up his nostrils, but now was clearly not the time to suggest that he used tissues rather than keep that sodden, infectious piece of cloth in his jacket pocket – not unless I wanted the fight to turn physical.

I patiently went through Bob's symptoms again. He didn't have a cough, he didn't have a temperature and he didn't have a sore throat, just a bunged-up nose. I'd already listened to his chest with a stethoscope and knew that there was nothing to indicate bronchitis; he just had a cold – man flu, I thought uncharitably. In reality, he didn't need to see a doctor at all, let alone require antibiotics.

At one time doctors did hand out antibiotics like sweeties but now we take the line of 'wait and see for five days' for most upper respiratory infections. We give antibiotics only if someone clearly has a chest infection (which we can hear when we examine them) or if symptoms persist. Sometimes, with switched-on patients who understand what we are trying to achieve, we give them a holding prescription, so that if they are not better in five days they can activate it. We stress, too, how important it is to finish the course.

More recent research done on tonsillitis and sinusitis (and ear infections in children) has shown that these, too, are caused by viruses and not bacteria, so that's why we adopt a wait-and-see policy with them, too. It's not because we don't care.

It was the over-prescription of antibiotics for simple infections that gave birth to superbugs such as MRSA, which resists most drugs and can cause appalling damage. I asked Bob if he was aware of this.

'The more antibiotics we give, the worse the resistance problem becomes,' I told him. 'So it's really important that we reserve antibiotics for nasty bacterial infections that really need them.'

He wasn't buying it. 'So you're trying to tell me that if you give me antibiotics now, then sometime in the future they may not work for me? Well, I don't care about that,' he said. 'What I care about is being able to get to a board meeting in New York next week and get a bigger budget for my team. And when I've had this problem before, my previous GP gave me antibiotics and I got better within a few days. Why on earth are you being so bloody difficult, doctor? Are you trying to save money or something?'

Antibiotic drugs were very cheap, so saving money for the cash-strapped NHS wasn't the issue. The point was trying to stop increasing resistance.

'Antibiotics are incredibly cheap. Honestly,' I pointed out, 'money isn't the issue here.' Unusually, I thought to myself, as increasingly what I am allowed to prescribe is governed by cost-effectiveness. 'It's antibiotic resistance that's the problem. And the chances are that, in the past, your colds would have cleared up just as quickly without drugs. Most infections get better within a few days.'

'Oh, for God's sake, Doctor Leonard, just because you're on the telly you think you can boss patients around. Just give me the bloody prescription and stop wasting my time.'

His time? *His time?* I had four patients whose appointments would now be late, not to mention my sick son, all because a not-very-ill, spoilt and portly man wanted some pills that probably wouldn't help cure his not-very-serious cold. Wasting *his* time was the least of my concerns. And anyway, why would a runny nose stop him going to New York? I'm sure there is space for a pack of tissues in business class.

I could feel my pulse rate rising, but getting angry wasn't going to help. I took a deep breath and tried a different tack. 'Do you think I enjoy this type of conversation?' I asked him wearily. 'It would be much quicker for me to give you the prescription you want – you would be out of here in a couple of minutes. But, the fact is, I don't think it would be in your best interests, so the answer is still no. Give nature a chance.'

Bob stood up abruptly and knocked the chair over. 'I'm fed up with this practice,' he said, wagging a finger at me. 'I spent ages yesterday trying to get through on the phone for an appointment. Now you've kept me waiting for more than half an hour, and what for? I'm going to make a formal complaint.' With that, he stormed out, slamming the door behind him.

Before I called in the next patient, I needed a breather. I made a quick call to check how Thomas was doing.

'Hi, Rosemary,' said Adrian. 'Do you want to speak to the invalid? I've given him some pasta and I've just looked in on him and he is fast asleep. He's still pretty hot, though. Shall I wake him?'

'No, don't do that – just tell him that I called to see how he was. Any other problems?'

'No, everything's cool – no worries.'

And I rarely did have any worries when Adrian was holding the fort at home.

When they got older, from the ages of twelve and fourteen, they were latch-key kids, but I had brought them up to be self-reliant and independent – just as my own mother had done with me and my sisters. Of course I felt guilty but, as always, it was a case of making what I hoped was the best compromise solution. I'm lucky that I really enjoy my work and it is an important part of my life – not just for the money, but for my own sense of completeness and self esteem.

For many years I raised them as a single parent and it was a pretty tough call. My marriage began to break down when my ex-husband's job in the engineering division of Unilever was moved to their main base at Port Sunlight on The Wirral, when the boys were four and six years old. As I was the main breadwinner, I stayed put in London and we both hoped my husband would get a job back in the London area so we could be a proper family again. Unfortunately this did not happen and the marriage didn't survive the long, enforced separations. However, after the break-up, my ex-husband came to London regularly to see Thomas and William, and they would travel north to spend weekends with him.

After the run-in with my antibiotics bully, Bob, I waited for his letter of complaint to arrive. I certainly never expected to see him again, since he had taken such a dim view of my medical expertise.

His letter didn't arrive, but when I saw his name on my list a few weeks later my heart sank. Was he desperate because all the other doctors in the practice had been fully booked up and I was the unwelcome last resort?

I buzzed through to reception.

'Has Bob asked for an emergency appointment? Last time I saw him he was less than happy. Did he try and book in with one of the other doctors first – I'd just like to be prepared if he's seeing me under duress?'

'No, he asked to see you specifically.'

That was odd. Maybe he was delivering the complaint by hand.

I called him in with some trepidation. I wasn't looking forward to seeing him again.

'Hello, what can I do for you?' I made absolutely no reference to our previous meeting.

'It's my stomach – it's swollen up like a balloon.' Yes, I thought very uncharitably and silently to myself, it's called fat. 'And I'm full of gas. I can't stop belching and farting. It's a real problem in meetings. They're such sombre affairs – but I can't seem to contain it. I'm becoming a joke.'

I asked him when the problem had started and if he could think of anything that may have triggered it.

'I can unfortunately,' he said. 'My firm took part in a huge dinner a week ago with one of the livery companies in the City. It was a wonderful meal, seven courses, all perfectly delicious, and we had lots of decent booze to go with it, including a few bottles of top-of-the-range Bordeaux. I've always had a healthy appetite and I know I over-indulged. I expected to suffer a bit afterwards, I always do, but I've never had after-effects like this. Usually any problem goes away in a day or two but this hasn't. I'd like some tests, Doctor Leonard, because it's really not normal for me.'

Although it was possible there could be something serious underlying Bob's bloating and burping, such as stomach cancer, it was highly unlikely. And he had only had symptoms for a week.

I took a deep breath. Yet again, he wasn't going to like what I was about to say.

'You haven't had your symptoms all that long. It's probably just excess acid from over-indulging. Why don't I give you something to reduce the amount of acid you are producing? I'm sure that's all you need – together with maybe a break from corporate entertaining.'

'Are you sure?'

'Yes, just give it a bit of time.'

'You keep a very tight rein on your prescription pad, don't you? And do you ever organise any tests? If all doctors were like you, Dr Leonard, the Health Service's financial problems would be solved, wouldn't they?'

I wasn't at all sure whether that was a compliment or a criticism, but he left promising, rather threateningly, to be back in a week if he wasn't better.

Two weeks later he was back on my list. Oh help, I thought, I'm in for it now. He's definitely going to demand tests and a referral.

'Hello, Bob, how are you?' I enquired, waiting for the tirade. 'How is your stomach?'

'My stomach's settled, though whether it was those capsules you gave me, or just laying off the claret I don't know. I'll soon find out, though – got a dinner next week.'

So why was he here? He hesitated before he started, and then suddenly blurted out, 'It's the mole on my back. My wife is worried about it. Can't see it myself, but she said it ought to be checked out.'

'How long has it been there? Is it itching, bleeding, or getting bigger?'

'No, I can't feel it. She says it's been there for years, and she's not sure if it's changed.' Uncharacteristically Bob seemed very ill at ease and displayed none of his usual bluster. I wondered why he was addressing the problem now. Was there something he wasn't telling me? Something more serious?

'Let me have a look.'

I took the opportunity while he was distracted removing his tie and unbuttoning his shirt to ask some more questions.

'You seem a little anxious. Anything else bothering you? Work OK? Are you being hit by redundancies in the City?'

'No, I'm a director,' he said proudly; 'my job's as safe as houses.'

An unfortunate simile given the economic climate, I thought, when houses were far from safe.

I checked his back. The lump concerned was really quite small and had no features to suggest it was anything other than a benign mole. I decided to do a little more digging and broached the subject of 'problems at home'.

Bob squirmed as he re-buttoned his shirt, cleared his throat, and fiddled with his tie. 'I'm a bit concerned about the old man.'

'Your father? What's wrong with him?' I asked.

'My dad?' he said, puzzlement creasing his heavily jowled face. Then he gave a nervous little laugh and his face reddened. 'No, no, nothing like that, my dad's deceased. It's my, er, my, er, penis. The thing is, I can't seem to satisfy the wife any more. It's difficult for her . . .'

'And for you,' I prompted.

'Yes,' he admitted, letting out a huge sigh, 'for me, too. The wife's frightfully sympathetic but that just makes it worse and it makes me angry with her, which I know is unfair. The more I try the more of a disaster it is. I'm thinking of moving to the spare room to save us both the embarrassment and humiliation. I realise it's probably normal to shut up shop sexually at my time of life. I've had a good run for my money so I probably shouldn't be complaining. I do enjoy sex, though, and I am going to miss it.'

I did my best to reassure Bob that he was right to be concerned and that at the age of fifty-six he certainly wasn't too old to enjoy a full and happy sex life. Now that he had stopped being enraged he had actually engaged my sympathy. I realised how difficult it must have been for him to confess to what he termed 'his loss of manhood'. One in ten men worldwide suffers from erectile dysfunction (ED) but only a third of them seek help because they are too ashamed or embarrassed. Which is a huge shame, but not only is ED behind the breakdown of at least twenty per cent of relationships, but it can also be a sign of severe, underlying medical problems, such as diabetes, low testosterone levels, and narrowed arteries, which also mean the man is at increased risk of heart disease. So it's taken extremely seriously by the medical profession.

'I got some of those little blue pills from the internet,' Bob told me. 'I waited for the magic to happen but nothing did. I had spent close to a hundred pounds on those pills and I had taken my wife to a Michelin-starred restaurant, hoping we could round off the evening in a romantic fashion when we got home. I even limited myself to one glass of wine with my meal. It was a disaster. Humiliating.'

'Sometimes those pills you get on the net are not the real deal,' I said. 'Many are fakes. There are plenty of charlatans around who will sell you rubbish and know that they can count on the fact that their customers will be too embarrassed to complain. It's much safer – and cheaper – to get Viagra prescribed by a doctor.'

'That's a relief,' said Bob. 'So I may not be a hopeless case. I read something about those scams in the *Telegraph*, that's why I thought I'd see you.'

Bob had loosened up a bit by now and confessed that on the two previous occasions he'd visited me he had actually wanted to ask about his ED but had bottled out the minute he entered my consulting room. So, I reasoned, all that aggression was due to inner anxiety.

I followed usual procedure and told him how common ED was and that in most cases it could be treated.

'We need to do some tests to check for an underlying cause,' I explained, 'because in older men it can be brought on by atherosclerosis, or hardening of the arteries, so I need to check your cholesterol and blood sugar levels, and I need to check your blood pressure.' The fact that he was overweight meant he was at higher risk of being diabetic, and probably had high cholesterol levels as well.

I also explained (with some apprehension, given his previous rants) that under NHS rules, initial medication had to be prescribed by a specialist clinic. I pre-empted another accusation about NHS money-saving by saying that this was a cost-cutting exercise that frustrated GPs, too. I said I was prepared to give him a private prescription for four Viagra tablets while he waited for his clinic appointment. At least, that way, he would be sure of getting the genuine article and, unlike many of my patients, I knew he could afford it.

His blood pressure was high – 160/100.

'What should it be, and what do those figures mean?' he asked.

'The top reading, the systolic, is the pressure the blood is leaving your heart, the bottom one, the diastolic, is the filling pressure. Ideally the readings should be a maximum of 135/85.'

'Is that why I can't get an erection? I didn't know that. I haven't got any other symptoms.'

'High blood pressure usually doesn't cause any symptoms,' I explained, 'and, no, it's not directly responsible for your erection problems. But, over time, it can cause damage to your arteries, which could contribute to the problem. It also puts you more at risk of having heart disease or a stroke. And you are not alone – it's an incredibly common problem. There are about sixteen million people in the UK with it.'

'So what do we do about it? I need pills, I take it?'

'Not straight away. We always do at least two readings before we start treatment, and the latest guidelines are that we measure your blood pressure over a twenty-four hour period, to be sure it's really high. It's possible it's high because you're sitting here in my surgery – no matter how nice I'm being to you.'

He smiled. 'The reason I come to you, Dr Leonard, is not exactly that you're nice – though you are usually. It's because you tell it straight. No beating round the bush.' Again, I wasn't sure if it was a compliment or not. 'You'd better tell me what I've got to do. I suppose the claret and the dinners have to go?'

'Altering your lifestyle will certainly make a difference.

Lose weight, healthy eating – you know, five good portions a day of fruit and veg, much less fat, cut down on booze.'

He pulled a face.

'Do you take any exercise?' I added.

'Well, I do the occasional round of golf. And walk to the station from home every day carrying a heavy briefcase.'

'How far is that?'

'Half a mile, perhaps less.'

'Not good enough,' I said. 'Half an hour a day brisk walking would be beneficial and would get your heart rate up – anything less won't help much. How about some tennis? Or do you have a gym near your office?'

'Well, yes, but it's full of much younger people,' said Bob. 'Some of my junior staff go there and I don't want them to see me huffing and puffing and looking ludicrous in a pair of shorts. Also, I work virtually twelve hours a day and I've no time for that.'

'I think your staff will admire you for trying to improve your fitness,' I said. 'You should try to make time for it if you value your health and your sex life. But don't go mad.' I had visions of him collapsing with a heart attack. 'Start gently, especially until we've got the tests done.' I did not want this obviously competitive man to keel over on a running machine or on a squash court after being inactive for years. 'Build it up gradually and get a properly qualified personal trainer to help you, if you can afford it.'

'And if I don't lose weight?'

'Then you'll need medication.'

'And I bet they have side effects?'

I gave him a really good – but honest – carrot to get his diet in order. 'One of the biggest problems with blood pressure medication is that they can cause erectile difficulties.'

'The gym it is, then.'

The blood tests confirmed that, though his blood sugar was normal and he wasn't diabetic, he did have a high cholesterol level. Again, changing his diet was an essential part of tackling this.

We agreed to meet up again in a month's time, when I would re-check his blood pressure.

Amazingly, he took my advice, though I'm not sure he would have done so if he hadn't got ED. I think that when I warned him that some blood pressure medication could make ED worse he realised that getting off his backside was a better option than sleeping in the spare room.

When he came into the room I could see he had visibly lost weight, which was quite an achievement after just four weeks.

'I'm watching what I eat,' he said. 'Or rather, the wife is watching what I eat. She is being very strict with me and stuffing me full of salad and fruit. I'm avoiding work dinners as much as I can and, when I do have to go, I'm learning what to avoid – like puddings and cheese. And I have actually joined a gym – I quite enjoy the exercise and find my brain's a lot sharper after a bit of a workout.'

'And the claret?' I asked.

'That's been the hardest bit. I've cut right back on that, too, though, and I suspect that is what is helping the most in shifting the extra pounds. I worked out that I was probably drinking at least five hundred calories a day. Now I have none during the week and just a couple of glasses at weekends. Might be another reason why I'm able to concentrate a bit more. And,' he added with honesty, 'all this has made me realise I was drinking far more than I should have been.'

The change of diet and taking more exercise alone had brought down Bob's blood pressure which meant he did not need medication for that. He did, however, need statins to deal with his high cholesterol. I discussed their possible side effects – mainly muscle pain – before getting on to the more sensitive subject of his erectile dysfunction. If I waited for him to bring it up I feared I might wait for ever.

'How is the ED?' I asked lightly.

Bob was still hellishly embarrassed and found something fascinating to stare at on his shoe laces rather than meet my eyes.

He cleared his throat theatrically and I let the silence run. Finally he said, 'Those little blue pills you prescribed are just the ticket. You just ask my wife. She was getting pretty fed up and I reckon you might have saved my marriage. But I haven't got an appointment yet at the hospital. You have referred me, haven't you?'

It was a fair question but, bearing in mind my previous run-ins with him, I was glad to see I hadn't forgotten and there was a copy of my letter to the clinic in his notes.

'Yes, I have. But, unfortunately, it's not exactly an urgent medical problem. You may have to wait a couple more months before you are seen.'

'Bloody NHS. Still,' he admitted, 'I suppose it could be said that a lot of this is of my own making. If I'd taken more care of myself in the first place this might not have happened.' He squirmed a bit and continued, 'I know I'm not an easy man, Dr Leonard, and that I've been rude to you sometimes, but I think you're a cracking doctor. No excuse for taking it out on you, when you have been so patient. I'd like to apologise for my bad manners.'

'That's very kind of you,' I said. 'People often get defensive and aggressive when they're scared or worried. Doctors get used to dealing with it,' I lied. I doubt I will ever get used to patients being rude or aggressive. I always find it upsetting, but coping with it, calmly, is part and parcel of being a GP.

CHAPTER SIX

HOSTAGE

I thought hard. And then harder still. No, there was nothing in my medical training about this. No tutorials about it when I was a medical student, and I didn't remember seeing anything that came close to this in any of my text books. My time working in a busy Accident and Emergency department? No. My year as a GP trainee? Nothing in that either. I was in completely unknown territory. I cursed the times I had thought a game of tennis was more important than attending a lecture. Fat lot of good a better serve and volley was to me now, if it meant I'd missed advice on 'Being imprisoned in a patient's home'.

The particular patient I'd been called out to see on that dark November evening was lying underneath a greying pink duvet. Seven years old, her eyes were wide open in apprehension and fear. Her mother was gently holding her hand. But the problem wasn't the patient – it was her father. He stood seething with anger beside her, staring at me.

'I'm telling you again, you are not leaving this room until you arrange for a paediatrician to come here and see my daughter.' Spoken with a thick African accent, his words were threatening.

I explained, for the fifth time, that it was impossible. 'If your daughter needs to see a paediatrician, then she has to go to the hospital. Honestly, that's just the way it works in the UK. GPs do home visits, but not paediatricians.'

Even if it had been justified, I honestly had no idea how I could get a paediatrician out to a council flat, especially at 9pm at night.

The girl wasn't particularly ill – she just had a cold and slight temperature – and it was questionable whether she even needed to see me, let alone a specialist. But by now that was irrelevant. Never mind whether she needed any medical attention – this was clearly a man who was used to getting his own way. I put my stethoscope away and shut my doctor's bag.

I tried to keep my voice calm.

'Really, there is nothing more that I can do. If you want your daughter to see a paediatrician then I can phone and arrange an ambulance to take her to hospital. And I'll phone the duty paediatrician so that the hospital are aware she is coming.'

I didn't add that I didn't think it was necessary. It wouldn't help an already tense, difficult situation.

I knew that both the ambulance crew and the paediatrician would take a dim view of such a waste of their time, and I'd have some explaining and apologising to do. But at that moment, I didn't care. I just wanted to get out of that room.

My offer of a fast ambulance fell on deaf ears. This man wasn't letting me go anywhere and, to ram the point home, he violently bolted the bedroom door. I looked at my watch and realised I'd been stuck in the flat for more than an hour. What was extraordinary was the way he was ignoring his daughter. He seemed oblivious to how his behaviour could be affecting her, especially as he apparently thought she was so ill. He didn't appear to be acting out of concern for her. He was just a bully, determined to get his own way. I had a suspicion that the fact that I was a woman was making matters worse – in his world women did as they were told.

I glanced at the girl's mother, who was sitting, quiet as a mouse, on the end of the bed. She looked terrified and I sensed this was not the first time she had witnessed her husband losing his temper.

Nowadays, any doctor in a similar position would hopefully be able to make a quick emergency call. But at the time, all I had was a bleeper that received incoming messages, and I had no way of letting the outside world know of my predicament. I was concerned about Thomas and William at home – I just hoped Adrian had put them to bed, and would hang on until I got back, whenever that might be.

I looked around the room. The flat was on the first floor of a large block built in the early fifties, and the walls were a dark dingy cream, and there was a thick layer of greasy filth on the old radiator. A brown patterned curtain half covered the window. A stale smell of fried food and musty clothes filled the air.

How much longer was I going to be stuck here? Did he intend to keep us locked in all night? I tried one more time with the offer of arranging an ambulance, to no avail.

'The doctor comes here. How many times do I have to tell you that?'

My fear was now being replaced by anger. I wanted to get out, and to get home. Keeping calm and reasonable hadn't worked, and a note of aggression came into my voice. 'Do you realise that you are holding me against my will, and that that is a criminal offence?'

'Don't tell me that,' he shouted. 'You are the criminal. You're not doing your job. Get a paediatrician here, now, to see my daughter. I'm not letting you leave until the paediatrician arrives.'

Out of the corner of my eye I noticed his wife slowly starting to move towards the window, at the foot of the bed. She caught my eye and beckoned me to come over, and slowly started to lift the metal catch, and push the pane open. This was madness – I dreaded what would happen if he spotted her aiding my escape. I was petrified his anger would turn to violence, and it wasn't clear who the victim would be. But if I was ever going to get out of here, I had to at least give it a try.

There wasn't time to think about how I was going to make it to the ground – I lobbed my doctor's bag out first and then took the leap of faith. I had no idea what I would land on. I was lucky – it was grass, and it was wet and soggy. Thank goodness it wasn't tarmac. My legs buckled as I hit the ground and I stumbled as I ran away from the scene as fast as I could. I didn't know if I was injured from the jump – the adrenaline blocked out my senses.

I went shaking back to my car, got in and locked the doors. My hand was shaking as I struggled to get the key in the ignition. I was petrified a large dark shadow would appear at the window, as I had assumed he would come after me. It seemed an age as the starter motor whirred and, as soon as the engine spluttered to life, my right foot hit the floor and the tyres screeched as I sped away.

I wasn't far from the surgery and I saw several office lights were still on – someone was obviously working late. I pulled into the staff car park. In fact, I don't think I could have driven straight home anyway – I was a jibbering wreck.

I was later told I was as white as a sheet when I walked in and that, combined with the mud on my clothing, immediately told my colleagues that something a little out of the ordinary had happened. I was put in an armchair, given a cup of coffee, and I told my tale. Next thing I knew, the other two doctors who had been doing paperwork were on the phone to the police. I was so tired and emotionally drained the last thing I wanted to do was make statements and fill in official forms. I just wanted to get home. But even then I could see there was a real principle at stake here – a doctor going out on a home visit should not be imprisoned in a patient's home. Not only that, but I was wondering what on earth had happened to the brave wife. I feared her angry bully of a husband was beating her up.

The police appeared remarkably fast and were fantastic. While a couple of kind and sympathetic PCs accompanied me home, several others went round to the estate, and (I later discovered) immediately arrested the father on a charge of unlawful imprisonment.

Despite the large shot of brandy comfortingly poured by Adrian, I didn't sleep very well that night. Not surprising, really – I don't suppose anyone would in the circumstances.

I certainly didn't feel like going in to work the following morning, but I knew my surgery was fully booked and if I wasn't there, it would only cause a lot of extra work for the other doctors. I also knew that often the best medicine for getting over a nasty experience is to get back to a usual routine as quickly as possible. So at 9am I was back in my consulting room, but I was desperately hoping I wouldn't have any awkward or demanding patients – my tolerance levels weren't going to be at their best.

The third patient I called had been added in as an urgent extra. A nine-year-old boy came in, followed by his mother, who was clearly more than a little annoyed with him. I wondered what the problem was. My question was answered by a stony silence. 'No, Jake, I'm not telling her. You can admit yourself how stupid you've been.'

He couldn't look me in the face, but rather mumbled at his knees, 'I've swallowed some magnets.'

I tried very hard to keep my eyebrows in their normal position.

'Errr . . . some magnets?' I asked. 'Just how many are we talking about? And how big were they?'

'About three, or maybe four,' came the whispered reply. 'But they're only the size of small marbles.' As if that somehow made it OK.

I had to ask, 'Was this an accident? Were they in your mouth and you just sort of . . . swallowed them?'

Silence again.

I looked at Jake's mother. 'Tell her, Jake.'

I was beginning to understand why she was so exasperated.

'I wanted to see if I could get paperclips to stick to my tummy.'

He'd been playing with a set of small round magnets and having fun making shapes with paperclips and other metal objects. It was the friend with him who had suggested they try testing the magnets' powers just a little bit more.

One swallowed magnet hadn't worked, so Jake had tried a second, then a third. Still no luck with holding paperclips in place on his skin. The experiment only came to a very abrupt end when his mother walked in.

Normally swallowing one small magnet does not cause any problems, as long as it hasn't got any sharp edges – but swallowing more than one is a different matter. The small bowel is usually more than two metres long, and coiled up in tight loops inside the abdomen. So if the magnets got separated, they could twist the intestine out of shape as they tried to stick together. Worst case scenario, the intestine could become so deformed it could become blocked.

I didn't need to tell Jake how foolish he'd been – his mother had clearly done that already. My job was to tell him the consequences of his actions, and what needed to be done next.

'You need an X-ray, as magnets will show up quite clearly. We'll be able to see where they are and, hopefully, whether they have stuck together in your stomach. And, if they have, it's likely they'll stay together. Your job,' I continued, 'is to check if, and when, they come out the other end.'

'Which means,' his mother helpfully added, 'that you've got to check all your poo. Very carefully.' There was a pause.

'I'll get you some gloves.'

Judging by the look on his face, it was the perfect punishment. He looked absolutely horrified.

Though potentially very serious, the incident brought me some much-needed light relief. Life was back to normal.

Well, nearly. I still had to face the prospect of the legal case connected with my imprisonment. I didn't relish the thought of going to court – quite the opposite in fact – but I had been brought up with a strong sense of right and wrong. That man needed to be taught that doctors could not be treated like servants, to be bossed around at his whim.

For a couple of months everything went quiet, and then, seemingly out of the blue, I had a call from my lawyer at the Medical Protection Society (MPS), the people who provide professional insurance for doctors.

'Rosemary, there is something you should know. The man in your case has taken out a charge against you. He is claiming you sexually assaulted his daughter.'

My jaw nearly hit the floor. 'He's what? Sexually assaulted his daughter? What exactly am I supposed to have done?'

My lawyer didn't have any specific details about the 'assault' and clearly thought the idea was as ludicrous as I did. It was obviously a plan rustled up by either the man, or his lawyer, to get me to drop my case.

The police and my legal team were determined I should press ahead and, under normal circumstances, I would have shared their view. But there was a complication, and it made me very scared.

I was aware that as I increased my work as a 'media medic' it put me in a slightly vulnerable position. To a large extent I agreed with the sentiment that if you put yourself in the public eye, or put your head above the parapet, then you could expect to get shot at. But a charge of sexual assault? Against a girl? Never, in my wildest dreams, had I envisaged that.

At the time I was working as the doctor on the *Sun* newspaper, the biggest-selling national daily in the UK. I had a suspicion that the man and his legal team might be starting a nasty, sordid and very public smear campaign against me.

I felt sure the *Sun* would not want their medical expert to be embroiled in something like this. As a single parent, the income from the column was helping to pay the mortgage I had taken out at the time of my divorce. This work was not something I could afford to lose.

There was only one thing to do. I had previously had brief conversations with the editor of the newspaper, Stuart Higgins, and had always found him to be a likeable man with a strong sense of responsibility over medical stories. I made an appointment to see him and told him the whole situation.

He was very understanding and advised me strongly that I should press ahead with my charges, that I should not be intimidated, and that *The Sun* would support me all the way.

Interestingly, once it became clear that I was not going to be frightened into dropping the case, the sexual assault charges mysteriously disappeared. It confirmed my suspicions – they were just trying to scare me off.

It took about eight months for the case to come to court. During that time I tried to forget about it as much as possible and continue with life as normal. We removed the family from our surgery list, as it was clearly impossible, under the circumstances, for either me, or any of my close colleagues, to look after them. I learnt soon afterwards that they moved out of the area. But, as the court date drew closer, I found myself having difficulty getting to sleep, I lost my appetite and shed at least half a stone.

I arrived at Middlesex Crown Court feeling tired and drained.

As I took to the witness stand, I kept reminding myself of my lawyer's advice: 'Remember, it's the defence lawyer's job to try and catch you out. Stay calm and just stick to the facts.'

It wasn't easy. My pulse was racing, and my palms were wet with sweat. As I had anticipated, the man's defence was that I had made the whole story up as a publicity stunt. But, thanks to Stuart Higgins' support, when I was asked about publicity I simply stated there hadn't been any. Not one word of what had happened had been printed in the national press.

Apart from his legal team, the man was on his own in court. I never spotted his wife or child, or any other family or friends for that matter. Under cross-examination, he came across as arrogant and self-righteous, and argumentative.

Thankfully, the jury did not take long to consider their verdict. They unanimously found him guilty.

In his summing up, the judge stated plainly that doctors need the protection of the law when they are going out and seeing patients, and it was totally unacceptable to hold me prisoner against my will. The man was sentenced to a twelve months imprisonment.

And the magnets? Jake knew, to his pain, when they came out, all three stuck together. I don't think that's something he'll ever do again.

CHAPTER SEVEN

TREE DOCTOR

As I woke up and mechanically thumped my shrill alarm clock into silence, I could hear the rain relentlessly beating on my bedroom window. I swore, tried to bury myself under the duvet and snuggled down for another couple of minutes. I'd had a couple of very early mornings that week doing stints on *BBC Breakfast*, and hadn't yet caught up on my sleep. I didn't want to get up.

The pit-pat of water falling on the window confirmed that last night's weather forecast, which had predicted heavy rain all day, had been spot-on. What joy. Not for me a nice dry, warm surgery – I had eight hours of home visits in the rain stretching out before me. I groaned.

Forcing myself from the warm bed, I walked to the wardrobe and surveyed my sartorial options. Looking smart was not one of them. This was a January day when a thick sweater, trousers, boots and my waterproof anorak were needed. I wanted to stay warm and, if possible, avoid getting soaked to the skin. In hindsight, I'm glad I put practical considerations first. Not only my tights but my reputation could have been damaged beyond repair if I had worn a skirt on that particular unforgettable morning.

Bent double against the downpour, I ran to my trusty little hatchback car and threw myself and my doctor's bag inside. When I turned the key in the ignition, the engine performed a few fainthearted turns before dying. I remembered that buying a new battery had been one of the many things on my 'to do' list, which somehow never got done. If I could only get it going, though, with a bit of luck the drive to the surgery should charge it up sufficiently for the day ahead. Finally I got lift-off and, with windscreen wipers going double time, I was on my way negotiating the narrow, suburban streets and one-way systems that baffled even the people who lived in them. Tree-lined avenues of semis became stark rows of terraces with the odd high-rise block towering above.

As usual, a cluster of patients were huddled in the porch of the surgery under the overhanging roof outside, smoking and looking bedraggled and miserable. I sprinted from the car inside as quickly as possible. Dumping my coat and bag in my consulting room, I headed off to find my stimulant of choice in the mornings – a cup of strong coffee.

The percolator was in the room behind reception and was always kept perked by Doreen or one of her staff. The door was ajar and I could see a line of wet patients, steam rising from their wet clothes, snaking round the waiting room waiting to be checked in for appointments or hoping to get one at the last minute.

After a couple of blissful sips, Doreen joined me and slumped into one of the threadbare armchairs opposite me. It was 9.15am and she'd been working since 8am. She dumped the large diary detailing the list of my home visits on the coffee table between us. Every surgery has its own system for dealing with these house calls. In some, they are shared out between all the doctors who carry them out after their morning surgeries. This has the advantage of doctors seeing the patients they know (and vice versa) but it also means that two of us can each end up doing the same long drive to visit two people in adjacent roads. One doctor doing them all can save a lot of time and that's how we operated.

Pouring herself a coffee, Doreen nodded towards the diary and rolled her eyes. 'Heavy day, Rosemary. It's what you would call a typical rainy weather diary. People are so lazy they don't want to leave their homes and get wet.'

My spirits sunk as I leafed through the list – two full pages already – and saw she wasn't exaggerating. There were so many visits requested that seeing everyone would be physically impossible.

'You can cut it down, though,' said Doreen. 'That Mrs Peabody, for example. Piles shouldn't stop someone walking to the surgery. And old man Wilkins, he can wait, too.' I trust Doreen's judgment implicitly, except when it comes to our Irish patients. Doreen's husband 'ran off' with a woman from Dublin and she has extended her prejudice to the whole of the Irish nation.

I poured myself a second coffee. Strangely, Doreen didn't seem in any hurry to leave, despite the queue outside.

'Busy out there?' I ventured.

'Lizzy can cope on her own for a bit,' said Doreen. She knew she had an experienced member of staff holding the fort, and I had a feeling she was waiting for something. Did she have a problem she wanted to discuss? She's a deep person, very good at hiding her feelings and unerringly professional in her work. I've never once heard her raise her voice on the phone in reception, despite immense provocation. Unfailingly courteous and polite, she always spoke slowly and reasonably. There was another side, though, one that she kept well hidden. I was once on the loo when the door to the Ladies thudded open and Doreen strode in, obviously enraged. Thinking she was alone, she smacked the wall so hard the cubicle wall trembled and her language turned the air blue. I learned some choice words that day before sheepishly sneaking back to my room. So if Doreen tells me I have to see someone, I'll obey; not just because she's invariably right but also because if I disagree it might activate her Attila the Hun side.

All the receptionists try to persuade patients to come into the surgery but, in the end, the decision isn't theirs to make. If a patient insists on a home visit, they have one.

Looking at the list, I could see the familiar names of housebound and elderly patients, whose requests were no doubt justified. But I wasn't so sure about the long list of babies and toddlers, let alone the twenty-three-year-old whose reason for requiring a visit was listed as 'aching all over'. I suspected that many of these people would have come to the surgery had it been a pleasant sunny day. I hadn't got time to see them all. I needed to phone some of them, in order to see which requests genuinely required visits and which could come to the surgery.

The first couple of patients on the list were about small children, who both had tummy upsets, so I arranged to see them. I knew that bringing a vomiting child to the surgery wasn't easy. But I managed to persuade the next two to come and see me the following day, having ascertained that there was nothing about their symptoms to set alarm bells ringing.

The next entry was unusual, not because of the patient's name, age, or even his medical problem. It was his address.

'Doreen?' I asked, puzzled, 'There's a patient listed here for a visit, but all it says for his address is The Old Oak. Is that a pub? I don't think I know it. I would ring him to get the rest of the address but it says there's no phone.'

A broad grin, verging on a smirk, spread across Doreen's face.

'I was wondering when you were going to notice that,' she said, a trifle smugly, I thought.

'Why?'

'It's not a pub, or even a house.' Even more smug now. The dramatic tension was killing me.

'Eh?'

'It's a tree.'

A tree?

'Yes, a real tree.'

'A tree? You're kidding me! You're saying I've got to go and see a patient who lives in a tree?' I checked the date – no, April the first was still months away.

'Yes, he's one of the protestors at the park.'

The light bulb suddenly lit up in my head.

There had been an application to raze a scenic, tree-lined ridge in the park to create an eighteen-screen multiplex cinema complex with restaurants, an amusement arcade, pubs, restaurants and the country's largest rooftop car park. Local people, furious that this unique space – so sacrosanct to family strolls, dog walking and joggers – was about to disappear, had mounted a furious protest and taken the matter to court.

The green lobby had objected because the open space was due to be destroyed. I opposed the new multiplex primarily because the local roads were already a nightmare and nowhere near capable of handling the vastly increased traffic the cinema complex would bring.

While the legal wrangling continued, the protestors arrived and set up camp in the two-hundred-acre park. They chained themselves to trees, erected tents, dug underground bunkers and constructed tree houses. They lived in the camp for more than a year, many of them for months at a time.

I tried to think this through logically. 'Does anyone know where this tree is?' I asked. 'Only there are an awful lot of trees in the park.'

Doreen replied, 'No, but the polite young man who rang said the doctor should go to the main bonfire area and ask where the tree was – someone will show you. The patient's not registered here, Rosemary, so do remember to get full details and a temporary resident form filled in and signed.' I was being reminded that even when you are up a tree it is important to complete the official paperwork properly. This never happened in *M.A.S.H.*

I did the urgent visits first and got to the park around lunchtime. The car park was some distance from the main protest site and it was still raining heavily. I zipped up my anorak and threw its flimsy hood over my head. Thomas, my eldest son, had lost his piano music, which he needed to take to school, and instead of eating break-fast I'd been searching round the house for it. I was incredibly hungry. Must learn to practise what I preach about that, I thought, and also make the boys take notice of my nagging about getting everything ready for school the night before.

I had only to follow my nose to find the bonfire because something that smelt gorgeous was cooking. I squelched and slipped through the sodden, sparse grass and mud underfoot, tightly gripping my doctor's bag, until I stumbled into a clearing where a huge pan of sausages and onions were browning in a pan over an open fire. A woman was turning the sausages and a man stood over her protecting the food from the rain with an umbrella. The aroma was delicious and my stomach rumbled. The sausages were a surprise – I suppose I had stereotyped the protesters and expected them to be vegetarians living on a diet of lentils and other pulses. I walked over to a young man who had just finished a sausage in a roll and was licking his lips contentedly. Rain was dripping off my nose by now and the anorak hood had become so saturated it was less than useless, I willed myself not to think about food.

'Hello, I'm the doctor – come to see... James, is it? The man who is unwell?'

'So good of you to come,' said the well-spoken young man as he extended his hand to shake mine, almost as if he were welcoming me to a dinner party. I held out my sodden, freezing palm.

'My name is Luke Sinclair. Could I tempt you to a sausage?'

My stomach grumbled in anticipation, but I felt I ought to see the sick patient first. 'OK,' he said. 'I'll try and save one for you. They're organic and totally delicious.'

'So, where can I find James?'

'I'm afraid he is up that tree,' said Luke, gesticulating towards a large oak behind me.

'Can't he climb down?'

'I'm afraid not. He's in absolute agony. Several of us have been up there to try to help him down but he can't move. If he does, he almost passes out with pain. We didn't want to do anything to damage him further so we rang your surgery.'

'So he's stuck up there?'

'I'm afraid so,' replied Luke.

Oh lordy, I thought. I do believe I'm going to have to climb up a tree.

Luke added kindly, 'James has never complained about anything in all the time he's been at the camp, which is why I'm taking this so seriously. I think he's really ill and we're all worried. He's a lovely bloke – totally committed to our cause.'

He'd need to be, I thought, as my eyes slowly scanned the tree. I had to tilt my head backwards into the full thrust of the rain and look up further and further until I could see some sort of wooden platform. The suspicion solidified – they expected me to climb this monster. I had to remain calm and show no fear. I was a doctor! Heights had never been a problem. Ladders were easy.

Twenty-five feet above, a couple of wooden pallets had been jammed into the space where the trunk split into three. A tarpaulin groundsheet had been rigged up on some overlying branches to give shelter from the rain, which was still tipping down, and which was now running down my back under my jumper. I blinked the rain out of my eyes and I walked over to the tree with Luke, who courteously held my elbow to stop me falling into the mud.

'James seems to have a severe, sharp pain in his tummy and is virtually immobile,' Luke told me. 'He is just lying on the floor up there, moaning.'

'How do I get up to see him?' I asked, confidently expecting them to have a proper metal ladder stowed away somewhere.

Sadly, they didn't. The only way up – or down – was via the sodden rope ladder I could see slapping against the trunk. Now this was going to be a challenge. 'It's best to go up sideways, monkey fashion,' Luke explained. 'The ladder swings about a bit if you try to use the rope steps like a conventional ladder.' I kept my expression professionally neutral but inside I had gone dead. How glad I was that my mother had persuaded me to join the Girl Guide pack she ran, because at least I had picked up a few survival skills. I was also hugely relieved that I was wearing trousers.

Although heights don't scare me, there was something unnerving and very uncomfortable about struggling up an unsteady, wet, rope ladder with large drops of rain dripping down my neck. I found it impossible to carry my doctor's bag because I needed both hands to hold the ropes – so I had to leave it with Luke. When I eventually reached the top, the only safe way to get off the ladder and on to the platform was on my knees. Hardly a dignified entry.

Tree Doctor

My patient, James, was twenty-four. I guessed he was probably about six feet tall but, as he was curled up in a ball, it was hard to tell. He was wearing faded, torn jeans, a stained, baggy, beige jumper and heavy leather hiking boots. He had four rings in each ear and one through his left eyebrow. His eyes, the colour of dark chocolate, eloquently expressed great pain. He lay on a grubby mattress with both hands clasped hard over his stomach, clearly suffering. Beside him was a rusty bucket and I could see that he had been very sick in it. 'Sorry about that, doctor,' he whispered, his anxious eyes following mine to the bucket. 'Not easy being ill up here, but so good of you to make the effort to see me. So appreciate it.' Suddenly his body jack-knifed and his features contorted in agony.

Trying to avoid looking at the drop below, I leaned over him, introduced myself and asked where the pain was coming from.

The brown eyes met mine. He told me, 'It started out in the centre of my stomach, but now it's spread to the right side.' He gasped, not moving his hands which stayed clamped to his belly. My first task would be difficult. I needed to examine him but this involved James uncurling so that I could see and feel his belly. I knew this would be exceptionally painful for him.

Although he winced, James bravely did what I asked and lay on his back breathing heavily, sweat beading on his temples while I felt round the area as gently as possible. I already suspected what the problem might be and the examination confirmed my suspicions. James was holding his abdomen very firmly and it hurt when I pressed it, especially on the lower right side. The real tell-tale sign was that the pain was worse after I released the pressure. That rebound tenderness made it highly likely he had appendicitis.

The appendix is a finger-like cul-de-sac attached to the end of the small intestine. Occasionally remnants of faecal matter can become trapped inside it, and the bacteria these contain multiply, leading to inflammation. The appendix then becomes full of pus and may burst. When this happens it can lead to inflammation and infection of the lining of the abdominal cavity – a condition known as peritonitis – which is potentially lethal if not treated. Sometimes the body's response is to create an abscess around the appendix to stop the infection from spreading. But that's nearly as serious.

There was only one course of action – James needed to go to hospital without delay. I whipped out my mobile phone from my sodden anorak pocket and rang 999.

'Hello, this is the emergency services. Do you require fire, police or ambulance?' asked the female switchboard operator with brisk professionalism. I should have remembered this was what they always asked. I did a quick mental calculation.

'I think I need all three.'

'Is that so?'

'Yes.'

'We don't like time-wasters.'

'I'm not a time-waster. I'm a doctor. It's difficult to explain.'

'Try me. But make it quick. We deal with genuine emergencies.'

'This is a genuine emergency. I have a boy with acute appendicitis stuck up a tree. He's in too much pain to be carried down. He's one of the park protestors. I need paramedics to treat him and take him to hospital, the fire service's hydraulic platform to get him down and the police to keep order. There have been clashes between the police and protestors in the past and I want to make sure it doesn't turn nasty.'

There was a silence that seemed to stretch for ever. Finally the operator grudgingly conceded.

'I'm on to it but if this is a hoax, I will make sure you are prosecuted. I've got your mobile number recorded.'

'Fine, you do that,' I said tersely, 'but just get me the help I need, please. This lad is really very ill.'

James managed a weak smile. 'Just what you need at a time like this – a jobsworth,' he said. 'I really appreciate what you are doing for me, doctor. Thank you so much.' He doubled in pain once more and his face turned so pale I feared he might faint.

'Take some big, deep breaths,' I told him. 'I think I convinced her. To be fair, she was only trying to do her job properly, and getting a man with appendicitis out of a tree probably doesn't cross her radar on a regular basis.'

I was aware of the large number of home visits still outstanding, but I wasn't happy to leave James until he was safely on his way to hospital. He was too ill. I shouted down to Luke to come up with my bag, and checked James's blood pressure while we waited.

'Is this the first time you've treated someone up a tree?' Luke asked when he arrived with the bag.

'Yes, and I hope it's the last time, too.'

James started to laugh but then realised it hurt too much.

'It's really brave of you to come up here,' he said. We tried to chat but James was too uncomfortable to talk, we were both shivering with cold and time hung heavily. After half-an-hour when there was still no sign of help, I began to think the operator had not taken me seriously after all.

Then I realised that I desperately needed to go to the loo. However, the nearest proper facility was at least fifteen minutes away and I wanted to be with James when the ambulance arrived. It was confession time. 'Sorry, but I need a toilet,' I said.

'Well there's the sick bucket up here,' said Luke, 'and we could both shut our eyes. It's a bit crowded, though.'

'Any other alternative?'

'There's a chemical loo to the right of the camp fire,' said James. 'You can use that – I'll be OK here with Luke.'

Tree Doctor

I had to brave another trip down the swinging rope ladder. It was worse than going up and I kept bashing my knees on the tree trunk. A crowd of protestors had gathered at the foot of the tree and one of them pointed out where the toilets were. I squelched across the mud to a white plastic hut where it took all my strength to open the warped and dirt-smeared door with my gloves on. It was not the sort of door you wanted to touch with your flesh. Even though it was cold and wet, the toilet stank so badly I felt nauseous. Somehow I managed to pull down my wet clothes and squat without actually touching the filthy seat, which must have been harbouring all sorts of germs. I tried to rinse my hands afterwards in freezing water from a water carrier but there was no soap. Today's health and safety police would have been horrified.

Soon after I'd made another rain-lashed climb to join James and Luke up the tree, the ambulance finally arrived. The paramedics spoke to the crowd of protestors gathered at the foot of the tree, shooting nervous glances upwards. A female protestor started screaming at them and I feared things were going to deteriorate. Finally a fit, young paramedic began climbing the rope ladder – he made it look easy. When he arrived at the platform, I introduced myself and explained the situation. I saw his features change from disbelief to acceptance and then genuine concern.

'We thought it was a hoax,' he said. 'We didn't take it too seriously.'

The makeshift platform was extremely crowded with four people on it and I hoped it was safer than it looked. The paramedic had to keep his elbows pressed tight to his body as he lifted his walkie-talkie to his mouth to convince his colleagues that they were dealing with a real crisis. If he had been in any doubt, a howl of pain from James swiftly dispelled it. I had to contort myself and crawl round the paramedic's body to feel James's pulse. His face was now the colour of parchment. This was getting urgent. 'It's more than a crisis – this boy's condition is serious, so get them to hurry up – please.'

Luke, teetering on the edge of the platform, said he could see a blue flashing light approaching through the trees. I leaned over and saw a police car below with a fire engine behind it. I could have screamed in frustration because I could see that they had turned up with a standard fire-fighting tender, with just ladders stacked on top. That wouldn't work – James was in too much pain to be carried down a ladder on a fire fighter's back. 'They haven't brought the bloody platform,' I said to no one in particular. The paramedic talked once more to his colleagues a lot less politely than I would have done.

'And tell the sodding fire brigade to get the doctor what she needs – we've a real sickie up here,' he shouted.

'He's not dying, is he?' said Luke alarmed.

'No, he'll be fine,' I replied with more confidence than I felt.

Eventually, an hour after I had made my emergency call, a behemoth of a truck arrived, with a hydraulic lift and cherry-picker platform on its roof.

The operator had a hard time weaving through the trees with this high vehicle, and many twigs and small branches were ripped off en route. When he reached the oak, the lift was slowly ratcheted up to the makeshift platform, crashing through branches and spraying lots of water onto the increasing crowd of onlookers below and onto us. I fervently hoped that it wouldn't crash against the platform when it reached it. Not only would that be agonising for James but the wooden pallet floor was merely wedged between branches and could easily become dislodged.

I had underrated the operator's driving skills, though. James bellowed in agony as on a count of three he was lifted with great care onto the cherry-picker. He found any movement agonising and made his descent slumped against the wall of the lift.

Once at ground level, the paramedics transferred him onto a stretcher and carried him to the ambulance through a crowd of curious and concerned protestors being held back by the police. I shinned down the ladder – I had the hang of it by now. Despite his pain before the ambulance doors closed, James had the courtesy to thank me again for my help, especially as it had involved climbing up a rope ladder. He even managed a weak grin. I didn't think he'd be volunteering for eco-protest duties again for a long time, committed though he was.

By this point it was almost 3pm and I still hadn't had lunch. As the ambulance sped off to the hospital, I was handed the sausage. They'd kept it for me, carefully wrapped in kitchen paper. It tasted wonderful.

I was aware that I still had a huge number of visits to do, but I reckoned I needed a bit of a clean up first. I trudged back to the car through the mud and headed for the surgery to try and dry off a bit before embarking on my other home visits, aware that I looked a wet, muddy mess. My hair was hanging in unattractive rats' tails beneath the saturated hood of my anorak. I was soaked through to my underwear and my hands were filthy with mud and god-knows-what from the foul loo.

Doreen eyed me up and down. 'I've seen you looking better,' she said.

'I don't suppose you'd look so great if you had climbed up a huge oak tree on a rope ladder to treat a patient,' I said.

'Wow. Was it genuine?'

'Yes. Life-threatening – for me as well as for him.'

'But you did get the form filled in?'

Of course I hadn't. I'd completely forgotten to fill in the temporary resident form for James.

Swearing under my breath, I knew that the first thing I had to do before I embarked on my remaining long-overdue home visits was to get everything written down. If not, there would be a comeback from the emergency services.

The remainder of the day was blissfully mundane and the most exercised part of my body on the twenty remaining visits was my hand as it wrote out prescriptions for painkillers and antibiotics. I eventually finished at 8pm but my much-wanted hot bath had to wait while I checked my sons had done their homework and music practice.

I received a copy of James' discharge summary from the hospital two weeks later. It confirmed that they had removed a burst appendix. After a week he'd been discharged back to his parents' home in Gloucester. A month later, I arrived for my morning surgery to find a huge bunch of flowers with an envelope attached and a generous token for a local organic butcher. Doreen was almost jumping up and down with curiosity but I decided to taunt her, said nothing, and took the gifts to my consulting room. Once there, I opened the envelope and unfolded a handwritten note. It read: 'With thanks and gratitude to my brilliant tree doctor. Hope you manage to enjoy some hot sausages. James.'

CHAPTER EIGHT

ROOTS

I had a rare free day and the spring sunshine was pouring into the kitchen where I ate an early breakfast and read the Saturday papers. The boys, teenagers now, were conforming to stereotype. They no longer did mornings and were still asleep or plugged into music. Feeling like a thief in the night, I put on my oldest jeans, T-shirt and over-sized sweater, opened the back door, slipped into my waiting boots and breathed in the sharp spring air. When April decides not to be 'the cruellest month' the weather can be glorious and I couldn't wait to get outside.

I inherited my love of gardening from my mother and now it is not only a fascinating hobby but therapy for me. Whether I'm digging, weeding, planting seeds, pricking out or hardening off, gardening imbues me with a rare, glorious sense of calm and the hours speed by far too quickly. When the boys were younger they would often stomp grumpily to the end of the garden or to the greenhouse to ask where their lunch was, because I had become so absorbed I'd lost track of time. Now they're older, it is they who will bring me a cup of coffee, or tell me that some pasta is ready in the kitchen.

I'd already done some initial preparation in my bit of London's heavy clay soil during rare, good-weather winter days, but now I was eager to dig some narrow trenches for my favourite vegetable of all – the Vivaldi potato. Yes, it is named after the composer, Antonio Vivaldi, because this particular spud is available during all four seasons. Developed in Leicester, it is known as the weight-watcher's potato because it contains fewer calories and carbohydrates than many other popular species. That's not why I grow it, though. It's because it makes such wonderful creamy mash.

I only managed a couple of hours digging and planting before capricious April reverted to character and the rain came pelting down. Unwilling to go in the house, I dashed for the greenhouse to start off some runner beans for putting outside a few weeks later after the risk of frost had passed, and to check on some early tomato plants I had grown from seed. Unfortunately, a good half of these had shrivelled up not long after producing their first seed leaves. When I shook them from their pots to perform a post mortem, I discovered that something had destroyed their roots. They hadn't stood a chance. It made me think of one of my patients called Alan. He had never stood a chance of having a happy and fruitful life either. What was done to him had been akin to taking an axe to the main stem that was so important to his identity; a blow from which he had never recovered.

When I first saw Alan at the surgery in 1990 I knew nothing of the terrible revelation that had torn his life apart. Most people love to talk about themselves but I had to prise every tiny personal detail from him. It was an exhausting business. His classic reply to any question was: 'Mustn't grumble.' And he never did, though he had plenty of reason to do so.

I saw from his notes that he was forty-five but he looked at least ten years older. He was slim to the point of emaciation and although I judged he was about six feet tall, his big shoulders were rounded forward in a stoop, which made him look far shorter. He had thick brown hair, with no signs of balding, but he was very pale, as if he hadn't been outdoors for some time. Dressed in a grey suit that had clearly seen better days, with a white shirt and dark green tie, it was obvious from his accent that he hailed from Yorkshire but I had no idea why or when he had moved to London.

He shook my hand politely, folded himself into the chair opposite and began to cough violently until his face turned red. No prizes for guessing what had brought him to the surgery then.

'How long have you been coughing?'

'Off and on most of the winter,' he told me. 'It's worse first thing in the morning. Sometimes it lasts for a good ten minutes.'

'Do you smoke?' I asked.

'I used to, doctor, but I gave it up a couple of years ago.'

'Well done,' I said. 'That will improve your overall health.'

'I didn't do it for health reasons, I'm afraid. The price of a packet of fags is out of my reach these days. I can't afford it but I still miss it.'

At my request, he shrugged off his jacket, unbuttoned his shirt and took off his vest, so that I could listen to his chest with my stethoscope. I could see that he had once been a physically powerful man because his shoulders and arms were over-developed and they still showed plenty of muscle tone. That was a bit of a puzzle because Alan's notes did not say that he was a manual worker but that he had a job in the civil service. He didn't look like the sort of man who would go to a gym either.

Initially I thought Alan had a chest infection, but when a course of antibiotics failed to get rid of it, I realised I had to explore other possibilities. I sent him for a chest X-ray and the results revealed hyper-inflated lungs and raised the possibility that Alan might be suffering from Chronic Obstructive Pulmonary Disease (COPD).

This condition was once called chronic bronchitis but that name was dropped because it is misleading and implies that an infection is present. COPD isn't an infection – it's permanent damage to the lungs. There is no cure, it destroys quality of life and is every bit as much to be feared as lung cancer.

With COPD sufferers the normal lung structure, which comprises tiny air sacs, is destroyed, which leads to breathlessness, while tissue lining the airways is permanently inflamed, which produces mucus and constant coughing.

Nine out of ten people who get COPD are smokers and those who smoke twenty cigarettes a day have a one in ten chance of getting it. There are three million sufferers in the UK, with another half a million people who have not been diagnosed. It accounts for more time off work than any other illness and is the reason behind one in eight hospital admissions. The average age of diagnosis is sixty-seven, so Alan was well on the younger end of the spectrum.

Alan didn't seem surprised that the lung function tests for COPD had proved positive. 'All miners get that in the end,' he said. 'I'd been expecting it.'

Miner? That was a surprise.

I hadn't realised that he'd been a miner because he had never mentioned it before and, besides, we don't get many of those in south London.

He wasn't being unduly pessimistic, though. Thousands of miners in the UK developed serious lung problems as a result of their work, which entailed breathing in coal dust every day. In 1998, the Department of Trade and

Industry settled a £7.5 billion compensation fund for miners affected by COPD.

I was curious about Alan's past life and said so. He told me, grudgingly, that he had left school at sixteen and gone down the pits 'like everyone else in our town. It was just what lads in our parts did and we earned a damn sight more money down the mines than doing owt else,' he said. 'It were hard graft, though, and we earned every penny.'

It emerged that Alan had spent the next twenty-three years working in a tunnel, lying on his back, often with his face only inches away from the coal face. He breathed coal dust into his lungs every working day. This would be a familiar tale to a GP working in a mining area, but for a southern city doctor it sounded like something plucked from a Victorian novel.

Alan told me he had come to London after the eighties' miners' strike, and the pit closures which had cost him his livelihood. He had retrained in Information Technology and got a civil service job in Whitehall. 'It did not pay well but I was one of the lucky ones, love, especially at my age,' he said. 'Many of my mates, who were nudging forty or thereabouts like me, have never worked again.' Then he abruptly changed the subject.

During the next few years, Alan's chest condition became gradually worse and he became a regular visitor. He was increasingly breathless and was seen both by me and the consultant chest physician who held a clinic at the surgery once a month.

Surgery staff usually get to know their regulars very well but Alan never opened up about his home life to anyone and always had an air of sadness about him. If I asked about his job he would reply that he was content or, if he was feeling really chatty, he would occasionally grumble about 'the management'. Unfailingly stoical, a typical response was: 'I've got a job, love, so mustn't complain. Plenty of people are worse off than me.'

One morning, a patient who knew about my love of gardening brought me some tiny beetroots she had grown from seed. I put them on the windowsill in my consulting room so they could continue to enjoy the light and so I would not forget to water them.

Alan came in, sat down, coughed for a few minutes, as usual, then his eyes alighted on the plants with interest. 'What are you going to do with those young'uns, love?' he asked.

This was the first time he had ever initiated a conversation with me. I was desperate to keep it going, so I told him about my garden. 'I started off growing herbs and salad stuff, such as cucumbers and tomatoes,' I told him, 'but although I grow leaves to put in salad I haven't had much luck with lettuces themselves.'

'You need to pick the right variety,' he said. 'Tom Thumb that you can eat all year round are good, or some of the "cut-and-come again" varieties. Give them plenty of muck to feed on and bolster them up and keep them wet.'

'The slugs target them mercilessly and always beat me to it,' I said. 'I've virtually given up, even though I hate to be beaten.'

'Aye. You need to forget all that organic stuff and declare war on them with a chemical,' Alan said with more emotion than I'd ever seen him display. 'Can't grow lettuces without slug pellets.'

'You know a lot about growing veg,' I said.

'Should do,' he said. 'I used to have an allotment in my other life, which kept us going in hard times. Now I've just got a window-box. I'll start you off some lettuces if you like, though, to see how you go.' Then his face, so briefly animated, sunk back into its usual frown lines as he watched me write out a prescription for more anti-biotics to deal with his latest chest infection.

Alan understood that there was very little that we could do about his COPD, other than try to improve his laboured breathing, but over the next few years he was stoical and never complained.

When I saw him as usual for his late October check-up and flu jab, Alan seemed even more reserved and mono-syllabic than ever. He was preoccupied, stared at the wall behind me a lot and I had trouble holding his attention. I decided to probe, in case another problem had developed. I knew that he had been forced to leave his top-floor flat because he did not have enough breath to climb the stairs. The lifts, he had told me, were always being vandalised and never worked.

'How's the new flat?' I asked.

'Just like the old one but on the ground floor in the same block,' he said glumly. 'It's better having no stairs to climb, what with my condition, but everything I try to grow in the window-box gets destroyed by local yobs, who have nothing better to do, or by the cats who use the earth as a lav.' He sighed heavily which led to a fresh bout of coughing.

'You OK, Alan?' I asked. 'Only you seem much quieter than usual.'

'Oh, I've just been a bit down recently, that's all. Bad time of year, what with the nights drawing in and being in the dark most of the time. But I'll be fine. It's nothing out of the ordinary.'

I tried to question Alan more but I could see that his mental shutters had come down again. 'You've got more important things to worry about than me, doctor,' he said. His chair scraped back and he got up abruptly and left without saying goodbye.

He was back in December, his cough worse than ever. After he'd sat down and drunk the water that I handed him, it still took him several minutes to find the breath to speak. 'Sorry to bother you, doctor, but I've got one of my chest infections again,' he told me when he was eventually able to talk. 'I've used up that emergency supply of antibiotics you gave me, but they haven't helped.'

This time Alan was in a very bad way and his forehead was clammy with sweat. He was extremely breathless and when I took his temperature I discovered that he had a raging fever. I listened to his chest and alarmingly heard nothing. There was normally a rattle caused by the underlying inflammation of COPD but this time the bottom of Alan's left lung was eerily silent, which pointed to one thing – pneumonia.

He needed to go to hospital.

He refused. 'I'll get MRSA, or one of those other nasty superbugs,' he said. 'I've read about how dirty our hospitals are now and I want no part of them. I've heard about people who have gone in and never come out. If I'm going to die, I want to die at home in my own bed.'

This was a bit extreme.

'Alan, you are not going to die – well, not yet, anyway. Not for a long time if I do my job properly. You've just got a nasty chest infection. If you go into hospital they can give you some intravenous antibiotics and you'll be home in a few days.'

'Doctor, I'm not bothered at all by dying. I just want to die at home.'

Alarm bells went off in my head. 'Do you think about dying a lot?' I asked.

'Oh yes, have done for years.'

The alarm bells got louder. 'Have you ever thought of harming or trying to kill yourself?'

'No, it's never been that bad. Anyway, I'm a bit of a coward. I could never do it.'

The other reason many people do not follow through on suicidal thoughts is that they realise how much it would hurt the family they leave behind. I realised that even after seeing him regularly for five years, I didn't even know if Alan had a wife or children. He had never once mentioned anyone close to him.

'What about your family, Alan?'

What followed next took me by complete surprise. Initially there was silence while Alan stared at the wall. Then I noticed his bottom lip begin to quiver, tears welled up in his brown eyes and this most reserved and taciturn character with the emotionless mask began to sob. My quiet Yorkshireman had fallen apart in front of me.

As he dabbed his eyes with a tissue I thought of the usual domestic scenarios that plunge people into such despair that they no longer consider life worth living. Had Alan's wife just left him? Perhaps my asking about his family had reminded him of the kids he had left behind in Yorkshire and hadn't seen for years. Perhaps his family had been killed in some catastrophe, such as a fire or road accident, or someone else he felt close to had just died. Could it be that his loved ones had been wiped out in a pit disaster? That would explain his preoccupation with death. I would never have guessed the truth, though, for I had always believed such stories were fictional and had no grounding in real life. Alan was still sobbing, so I clasped one of his hands and offered him more tissues from the box on my desk.

'Alan, please tell me what's wrong. I'm here to help you.'

And then, bit by bit, the whole dreadful story came out.

Alan had come from a large mining family in a small Yorkshire town. His father, who had also been a miner, died prematurely in a pit disaster when Alan was seven years old and his widow and her nine children lived mainly off the compensation until they could go out to work and help their mum. Alan had come along five years after the other kids. He had shown promise at school but no one expected him to do anything else than go down the pits as his brothers and father had done before him. Alan's wages were too badly needed by his mother for further education to be an option. He had a sister, Margaret, who was sixteen years older than him. 'I don't remember much about her,' he said. 'Before I was five and starting school, she and my mother had already badly fallen out. She met some fellow from Glasgow and moved up to Scotland. We never saw her again and when she sent Christmas cards or a birthday card for me, mum would throw them in the fire. I didn't dare ask why.

'Because I was so much younger than the other kids they called me the mistake,' he said with a bitter laugh. 'I didn't realise then how much of a mistake I really was.'

Alan got married when he was twenty-one. 'She was a nice enough lass,' he said, 'but a bit lightweight, if you get my meaning. She was always spending my money on catalogue clothes she didn't wear. She always wanted the latest washing machine or TV, even though the old ones hadn't worn out. She liked keeping up with the Joneses, did our Moira.

'We didn't have much in common. I'm a simple man and as long as there was food on the table and I could escape her nagging by going down to my allotment and tending my veg, I was reasonably content. It might have helped if we'd had kids but it didn't happen for us. I'd never have left her, doctor, but then the strike came along and that changed everything.'

During the months when the miners were out of work in the eighties there was incredible hardship in towns like Alan's. Because he and his wife did not have children, they were not in the front line to receive financial help from the union, so they plundered their savings to survive. When the money ran out and they could no longer pay the rent on their small terraced house, they moved in with Alan's mother before the bailiffs could take away their furniture.

'Moira lost her job – no one had any money to spend in the butcher's where she worked – so the three of us were stuck together all day and every day. Mum, living on her pension, hinted that we had become a burden and she 'wanted her home back'. I knew that if she and Moira had got along better, perhaps she wouldn't have reached the end of her tether like she did. But she and Moira rowed about everything, from which TV programme to watch to how long we were allowed to run the immersion heater before having a bath. I'd come back from the allotment and Moira would be in the bedroom crying and complaining about something my mum had said or done, and I would get an earful from Mum about Moira being unreasonable and spoilt and never helping her. I dreaded going home – but that had an "up side". I had a bumper crop of vegetables that year and even managed to sell some to help out the family finances.'

On one particularly bad day, when there was no coal left for heating and no money remaining for food, Alan's enraged and frustrated mother screamed at him the words that stole his life: 'I wouldn't mind so much if you were really my own son.'

'I can't tell you how those words froze my heart,' said Alan. 'I was in a fog. I thought I'd misheard but she repeated them and I knew it was the truth. Every snigger during my childhood, those looks the family shared which I did not understand . . . I wanted to scream.'

He didn't, of course. Alan balled his fists to contain his rage, then went and sat in his allotment shed until he was sure his wife and the woman he had known as his mother had gone to bed.

The next day, he sent his wife out on an errand and told his mum that she owed him the truth and that he would not budge from her kitchen until she came clean. It emerged that his 'mum' was really his grandmother. His mother was the person he had known as his oldest sister,

Margaret, whom he could barely remember and with whom the family had lost all contact.

'Mum told me that Margaret had become pregnant with me after a very brief fling during the war with an American GI stationed on the airbase in the next village,' he said. 'He flew on missions to France, was reported missing, presumed dead, and Margaret never heard from him again. She didn't even know his surname.

'The most important thing for my mum was that no one in the village should know that her daughter had a baby out of wedlock and I despise her for that. In those days, unmarried mothers were regarded as a disgrace and Mum and Dad wanted to hush the whole thing up. Margaret was packed off to an auntie's in Scarborough and Mum faked a pregnancy.

'After I was born, Mum told everyone that I was hers. People may have had their suspicions but no one actually knew the truth. Margaret, when she came home from her auntie's, was told to keep her mouth shut if she wanted to continue to live at home. It was all brushed under the carpet and never talked of again.'

'Did no one try to trace your father?' I asked. 'He might have survived or he might have had a family who would want to meet you.'

'What, and risk the truth coming out?' said Alan. 'My family didn't try. And Mum made life impossible for Margaret – I don't blame her for leaving, though I wish she'd had the courage to take me with her.'

Alan said his real distress came not only from the way the news was broken but from the fact that it had been hidden from him for so long. All his life the people he had known as Mum and Dad were nothing of the sort. 'They kept quiet for forty years. Why didn't they tell me when I was young? Didn't they think I had a right to know who I was? I was a mistake, all right, that's all I meant to any of them.'

The fragile house of cards that was Alan's family life fell apart at that moment. His relationship with his grandmother/mother was fractured beyond repair and his wife, intolerant of his increasing broodiness, told him that she had met someone else and was leaving him.

Alan moved out of his mother's house soon afterwards. He could never make her understand how betrayed he felt and she persisted in saying that she had acted for the best.

'For her, maybe, but it wasn't for my best,' he said bitterly. 'I spoke to my other brothers and sisters but they didn't seem at all bothered – or even surprised. They had all been party to the secret but Mum had sworn them to silence. Her word was law in our house. When one of my brothers actually told me that it was time to "move on" I whacked him. I'm normally a very calm man and this frightened me – I knew I had to get out or go mad. I got a job here in the south and left without saying goodbye. I've never been back and I never want to see any of them again.'

Now, with no one to care for him and coping with a debilitating illness that woke him at night and stole his breath, Alan was a terribly sad and lonely soul. No wonder he thought so often of death.

I was aware by now that I'd been with Alan for much longer than the ten minutes allotted for each appointment and that there would be a queue of irritated patients building up in the waiting room. Although I wanted to talk to him for longer, I knew that it just wasn't possible.

Alan remained adamant that he would not go into hospital, so I gave him antibiotics and made him promise that he would call the surgery if his breathing got worse. I also added him to my list for next day's surgery so I could check on his physical state and try to address his fragile mental one. I also made him promise to return.

'If you don't, I'll come round to your flat and get you,' I warned him, and was rewarded by a faint smile.

Alan refused to take anti-depressants but surprisingly he did agree to see the practice counsellor. I'm a great fan of 'the talking cure' and apart from being highly skilled, counsellors can give patients the one thing I often find impossible – plenty of time. We both raised the issue of tracing Alan's real father but he saw no point. 'It might be possible, I suppose,' he said. 'Someone must know something about the airmen who were stationed near us, but what if he didn't survive the war? That would be more bad news that I don't want to know. I might not be able to cope with another loss now. And if he survived he's probably got a family of his own. The last thing they'll want is me appearing in their lives. I don't want to be rejected again.'

I could see his point.

There were no happy endings with Alan's estranged family either. No matter how much the counsellor and I pushed for a reconciliation that may have helped Alan come to terms with his past, he said that he would never forgive his family for the cover-up. It was his decision and we had to accept it. He refused to budge.

Alan has retired now and his chest is worse, but he seems to walk a little straighter, as if talking about his hurt has lifted a weight from his shoulders.

He still sees me regularly and gives me young lettuces, and I've followed his advice and chemical warfare against the slugs means I now get a decent crop. When he started to bring lettuces to every appointment, I suspected that Alan must be growing them in something bigger than the window-box of his flat.

'You really must stop doing this,' I told him. 'You'll have none left for yourself.'

'Don't you fret, doctor,' he said, his mouth almost creasing in an approximation of a smile. 'I put my name down for an allotment after I saw your little plants that first time. I realised how much I missed growing things. I got my plot nine months ago, hired a digger to get the land in order, bought a pile of manure, and I've been growing vegetables on it for the past six months. My marrows are so good I may even enter them in the local produce show. You've got the same sort of soil in your garden as me, so what vegetables do you think work well here?'

'Since my sons have grown older, I've expanded my vegetable repertoire,' I told him. 'I've got broccoli, peas, mangetout, runner beans and broad beans in raised beds. I'm also a big potato fan, particularly the Charlotte and Vivaldi varieties.' I swear Alan's eyes went misty.

'The Vivaldi,' he said with awe. 'Now there's a wonderful spud – it's one of my favourites, too. So if you ever run out, you know where to come. I always make room for those beauties.'

I noticed that although Alan's cough was worse than ever, his complexion was no longer so pallid and I remarked on it.

'I'm out in the fresh air more because of my allotment,' he said. 'And there's a nice bunch of blokes there. Most of them are escaping their wives, if you ask me, so I count myself lucky I don't have one. I can stay on my plot as long as I like and know I won't be nagged for it when I get home. I've built a little shed up there and take a thermos of hot water with me so I can have a cuppa when I like. Living alone isn't all bad news, doctor, and I'd rather do that than endure a life sentence with someone I couldn't abide. I tried that once.'

Alan now brings me plastic bags full of the seedlings he has harvested from his crops or small starter plants. His breathing is slowly getting worse but he does seem less withdrawn and genuinely pleased to see me.

Doctor, Doctor

After all those years of stilted silences, I do believe that for the first time in our long relationship, my sadly silent Yorkshireman and I have at last found common ground.

CHAPTER NINE

A QUESTION OF SEX

GPs are just as human as anyone else. Though I've been doing the job now for more than twenty years, like every GP I still make mistakes and I'm still learning.

Jean is a typical illustration of this.

I'd known her for several years and, at the age of eighty-three, it had become apparent that she was suffering from increasing memory loss. This had been diagnosed several years previously as due to early vascular dementia. Different to Alzheimer's, this happens when blood vessels in the brain become clogged up and it results in a gradual loss of blood supply to the nerve cells in the brain.

Jean lived alone in a sheltered-accommodation flat. She had married a serviceman in her teens but had been widowed in her early twenties when her officer husband was killed on active duty in Korea. The couple did not have any children but Jean told me that she'd never felt the need to remarry.

'I have plenty of male companions,' she said with a girlish laugh and I nodded patronisingly, imagining bingo or whist sessions and cosy coach rides to the coast with an OAP club. No one in the surgery, including myself, bothered to inquire about her 'current relationship status', as we primly call it. We all assumed that at Jean's age she was long past having sex.

Despite her cut-glass accent, Jean dressed eccentrically and was always heavily made up. A yellowy-brown foundation cream caked every wrinkle in her face, blue eye shadow was liberally applied to the lids of her deep-set eyes and she had sought to make her thin lips appear more plump by painting on a lurid red lipstick complete with a cupid's bow. Brown crayon made shaky curves where her eyebrows had once been and her hair was dyed a yellowish blond.

Jean was into layering well before it became fashionable but clashing skirts, tops, coats and shoes always made her look like a rainbow on the move and she wore so much jewellery she clanked as she walked. Her fingernails were invariably painted and she always sported lace fingerless gloves, in a variety of colours, which looked as though they needed a good wash. I have never seen anyone go to so much trouble to look so ghastly.

The first hint that Jean's problem might be due to something more than dementia arose when a member of

the local church came in to the surgery to make a doctor's
appointment. Doreen said that she had specifically asked
to speak to me because I was a friend of Jean's.

'Something's up,' Doreen warned me before I buzzed
this mystery patient through. 'She's a skinny, little woman,
so I don't think she's got enough power in her arms to
do you any harm, Rosemary, but she looks mighty angry
about something. I could get someone to loiter outside,
if you like. I don't reckon she's any friend of Jean's
herself.'

'I'll take my chances,' I said.

Initially, when the woman, whom I had never met, sat
down in my consulting room, she seemed hugely embarrassed as well as furious. She held her large handbag in
her lap like a shield and gazed through the window with
pursed lips, virtually hyperventilating, obviously preparing
a speech.

'What seems to be wrong?' I inquired.

'Nothing's wrong with me,' she snapped. 'It's that Jean.
The one who sees you.'

Whatever Jean was guilty of, I'd obviously been tarred
with the same brush.

I forced a smile, then embarked on my well-honed spiel
about confidentiality and not being able to discuss another
patient. The woman stood up, slapped my desk aggressively
and leaned over it.

'I will have my say,' she told me, jaw jutting, eyes hostile,
spittle flying so far it hit my face.

'OK,' I replied, 'but please sit down.' And, I thought silently, please keep your saliva to yourself. I'm exposed to enough germs in this job without you spraying my body with any more.

Reluctantly, she complied, smoothed her wool skirt over her bony knees and began, keeping her eyes down.

'We all know Jean's not right,' she said, 'and we've all tried to be kind and understanding.'

She looked up and I nodded encouragingly, glad that we seemed to be in calmer waters.

'She goes to the same church as me,' continued the woman, 'and after the service we all bring in cakes to eat and share. We take it in turns to make the tea. It's a bit of a get-together – a chance to catch up with people.'

I nodded, wondering where the monologue was going. Normally, the longer the lead-in, the worse the problem. 'Well, this Jean never brings anything to eat but she scoffs all our stuff,' continued the woman.

I was about to interrupt, thoroughly irritated, when she started again, this time speaking at double the speed. 'I wouldn't mind that so much but she's all over the men – she plays up to them like some floozie. Mostly they laugh it off, but I've heard plenty of tales. This time she was after my own husband, Bill. She told Bill that if he wasn't getting any . . . you know what I mean, doctor, the sacred thing between a man and wife . . . that he was always welcome to come round to her flat and she would see him all right. She's made plenty of other disgusting suggestions to other husbands and respectable widowers, too, but I really couldn't repeat them to you, doctor. She's got a filthy tongue on her underneath that hoity-toity voice. We wives want her stopped.'

Although I nodded sagely and made sympathetic noises, I found it difficult to keep a straight face while this uptight and prudish woman painted a picture of eighty-three-year-old Jean as a shameless Jezebel. Despite probing her for more details, the woman wouldn't tell me what Jean had been saying to the men because 'it was too rude'.

'What do you expect me to do?' I asked. After all, I was a medical doctor, not a marriage guidance counsellor, and I could hardly turn up at the after church get-together and tell Jean to shut up.

'Have her locked up, stick her in a loony bin where she belongs,' hissed the woman. 'Put her away where no decent man can be tempted by her dirty talk. She's loose, that's what she is.'

'I'll speak to Jean,' I assured her, a little falsely. After all, what was I supposed to say? And, anyway, was it really a doctor's business if one of their patients was a flirt? But I had to tell this woman something to get her out of my room.

'Make sure you do,' she said darkly as she left. 'I've said my piece.'

At the next practice meeting I couldn't wait to tell the other surgery staff about the conversation. Everyone knew Jean and realised she was a bit batty. But was she really a femme fatale in bag-lady clothing? It hardly seemed likely. None of us were sure what to make of it or what, if anything, we could do. And anyway, we only had one woman's word for Jean's behaviour – and we didn't know if she was telling the truth or not. When in doubt, do nothing. So that's what we did.

A couple of weeks later, Jean came into the surgery.

She had only just reached the reception desk when her problem was broadcast to all in hearing distance.

Lizzy was manning the desk and was on the phone as Jean arrived.

'Hello, Lizzy, I've got terrible thrush. The discharge is awful . . .'

'Jean, just wait a minute. I'm on the phone.'

But Jean didn't wait, so the poor patient at the other end of the line trying to make an appointment was treated to the graphic details, as well as everyone in the waiting room.

'But it's green and smelly; really very unpleasant. I really think I ought to see a doctor today.'

'Jean, just let me deal with this person on the phone.'

Everyone in the waiting room hastily retreated behind the covers of their books and magazines, hiding their faces while pretending not to listen to every unsavoury detail. Lizzy did her best to shut Jean up and explained that intimate details were best discussed behind closed doors with the doctor. Thank goodness for Lizzy's endless patience and good nature. She had started working for the surgery when her youngest child, who has now just left university, went to secondary school. She split her time between the notoriously hectic reception desk and doing paperwork in the office upstairs. She reckoned that getting away from reception kept her sane. 'If I was there all the time I'd lose my rag with some of them. They can be so demanding, not understanding the pressures we're under. As it is, I'll do my four-hour stint, then escape to the office where it's a bit calmer, and where no one can shout at me if they can't get an appointment.'

Lizzy buzzed me through when she saw I was free.

'I know it isn't an emergency, but is there any chance you could fit Jean in this morning? Otherwise the whole of south London is going to hear about her vaginal discharge.'

Jean continued to treat her audience to a blow-by-blow account of her complaint while she waited for me to summon her. She seemed to have completely lost her sense of embarrassment – for herself and everyone else.

She was her same cheerful self when she came into my room. She told me what a lovely place I had, as she always did, admired the plant on the windowsill and complimented me on my lilac sweater.

'I used to have one like that as a girl,' she said. 'Happy days.' Clearly in the mood for a chat, it was difficult to pin her down to the reason for her visit.

'Jean, Lizzy tells me you've been complaining of a vaginal discharge. How long have you had it?'

'Oh, not long, doctor. Just a few days. It's so unpleasant. Please do something.'

Thrush is very unusual in an eighty-three-year-old and my immediate thought was that she had a tumour somewhere in her genital tract. I needed to have a look.

Jean stripped off her numerous layers of clothing, along with some truly filthy underwear, and lay down on the couch so I could examine her. She was right about the discharge. Something nasty was going on. I took swabs, gave Jean antibiotics and said I would arrange for her to have an urgent ultrasound scan of her pelvis. But before any results came back, another 'concerned local resident' came to see me. This one seemed much more reasonable.

'I've known Jean for years and I know she's a patient of yours,' she began.

'I can't discuss my patients,' I told her.

'Yes, I realise that,' she continued, 'but this is serious. Something is very wrong with her. Her behaviour has changed.'

I waited, assuming she would just confirm what we had witnessed in the waiting room. But what she was about to describe was a different type of behaviour.

'She stands outside Tesco most evenings and when she sees a man on his own she approaches him with her trolley . . .'

'Yes . . .'

'She asks him if he'd like to come back to her place for a bit of, a bit of – sexual intercourse.'

The woman was red in the face by now, arms crossed over her chest.

'How do you know she does that?' I asked.

'She propositioned a friend of mine. He'd seen her approach several other men. He wasn't sure what to do, so he came and told me.'

Again, when we discussed it, my colleagues and I attributed this brazen behaviour to Jean's dementia, which appeared to be getting much worse. But one of the doctors, David, had a different take on the matter. Quietly spoken, handsome and extremely efficient, David has a talent for administration, is extremely confident and is always chasing me to catch up on paperwork, which I realise is important but which I nevertheless find deadly dull. I grudgingly have to admit that he is firm but fair.

David also has an amazing head full of medical knowledge, facts and figures. If I ask his advice, I know I will get an answer based totally on facts or probability, rather than one that comes from an emotional or self-interested point of view, and he has often enabled me to see something from a different perspective. When he asked if he could see me after the meeting, I assumed that he wanted to remind me about some paperwork I'd forgotten to do, but I was wrong.

'I've been thinking about Jean ever since she was discussed at the first meeting,' said David. 'My maternal grandmother was a randy old dear and, apparently, at the country house parties she used to attend she had a quite a reputation for bed hopping. My mother believes she screwed my grandfather into an early grave.'

I laughed.

'You wouldn't have believed it to look at her,' continued David. 'She was very proper, a real lady, but she had a huge libido. It made me wonder whether Jean is like that, too. What if she is a lot more sexually active than we think? Perhaps some of those men do take her up on her offer and she has a sexually transmitted infection, which she may now be passing on to the church congregation, Tesco shoppers and anyone else who takes her fancy. The men who say yes are hardly likely to tell their wives, are they?'

I had to laugh, but he had, as usual, made a very valid point.

When Jean's swab result came back, it showed David was right. Again. Jean had trichomonas vaginalis (TV for short) – a sexually transmitted infection (STI) which often goes hand-in-hand with gonorrhoea. So much for my assumption that Jean was sexually inactive. This was just my first wake-up call.

I rang Jean and asked her to come back to the surgery for treatment and more tests. When a patient has TV they often have gonorrhoea as well – I needed to take another swab. Like many patients with memory problems, Jean often missed appointments and it took three attempts, even with Lizzy phoning and reminding her beforehand, before I eventually saw her again. When I did, she was her usual upbeat self and as uninhibited as ever.

'Jean, you have an infection. You need antibiotics.'

'What type of infection?'

'It's an infection called trichomonas.'

'And how did I get it?'

I should have been more prepared for this. It wasn't going to be easy. When I broached the subject of sex, I tried to be respectful and tactful, because many people, especially older ones, can become embarrassed. Jean, however, wasn't one of them. When she realised what I was getting at, she laughed delightedly. 'Do say what you mean, Dr Leonard. I've always enjoyed having lots of male friends and I love going to bed and having nookie with them. Some of the poor old souls don't get sex any more and it does them a power of good, so what's wrong with that?'

'Nothing at all,' I replied. And I meant it. I've always been in favour of women enjoying active sex lives, no matter what their age, so that didn't faze me. What did faze me, though, as the conversation continued, was the sheer number of men involved. Even Jean herself had lost count. 'Probably a thousand,' she ventured. 'Perhaps two thousand? Who's counting? I've really no idea. Please don't ask me to name them, Dr Leonard, I've got a terrible memory these days and I don't keep an appointments' diary anymore because I always lose it.'

I asked Jean if she used any protection and she looked at me as if I were barmy. 'I took precautions when I was younger, of course,' she said, 'but after I'd gone through the change of life there didn't seem to be any point. I couldn't get pregnant and I hate all that fumbling around with rubber – men are so inept at putting the things on. I did once try a Dutch cap but it meant rushing off to the bathroom to cover it with cream just when you were in the mood – was a frightful bore. In the end, it rotted through lack of use and I threw it out. That was decades ago.'

Jean was absolutely clueless about STIs. She thought that only young girls or gay men could 'catch the clap' by having sex.

'I'm in my eighties, doctor, my body has fought off everything going by now. I'm not going to get something like that at my age.'

'But you can, Jean, and you have,' I told her. 'You can also pass it on to your gentlemen friends and they will all become ill, too.' I had an image of an epidemic – the whole of the female congregation of the church, along with all the wives of Tesco's male shoppers, descending on my surgery en masse brandishing their rolling pins because they had caught an STI from their husbands, who had all engaged in a romp with Jean.

'It's important that you don't have sex till the infection has gone.'

Jean turned truculent and defensive. 'If you think I'm going to stop having sex with my gentlemen friends, young woman, then you must think again,' she said huffily. 'We enjoy it and it does no harm. And I suppose because you are giving me antibiotics you're going to tell me I can't have a glass of sherry either.'

There is a widespread perception that you can't drink alcohol while taking antibiotics, and it's just not true. For most antibiotics there is no problem washing them down with booze, along as you don't drink so much that you forget to take the tablets. But there are a few exceptions. Metronidazole, the treatment I was giving Jean, was one of them.

'Alcohol won't stop the treatment working, but the combination might make you feel really sick. I wouldn't advise it.'

'Well, you're being a complete killjoy today, Dr R.'

I calmed her down, took more swabs and sent them for analysis. The results revealed that not only did Jean have TV, but chlamydia and gonorrhoea, too. I prescribed treatment, but I clearly needed to get expert help. It would be a horrendous job trying to trace all the men Jean might have infected, especially when she could not remember their names. Should we get something read in church or put up a notice outside Tesco's telling men who had enjoyed sexual relations with Jean to contact us in the strictest confidence?

Far from being aghast at the latest diagnosis, Jean regarded her raft of STIs as a badge of honour.

'Well I never,' she exclaimed gleefully. 'Fancy that – me, a woman in her eighties, getting a dose of the clap. I never would have believed it.'

Me neither, I thought. That had been the problem.

Getting Jean to cooperate in the next stage of her treatment – going to the local Genito-urinary Medicine (GUM) clinic required enormous perseverance on the part of virtually everyone in the surgery, especially Lizzy, who had a soft spot for the eccentric elderly lady. Again, Jean kept forgetting appointments. Her memory was clearly getting worse, along with her increasingly uninhibited behaviour. She had loudly broadcast to the occupants of the waiting room on the day I saw her that: 'Doctor Leonard thinks I may have a sexually transmitted infection – isn't that rather fun at my age!'

At the GUM clinic Jean had all the standard tests and received yet more treatment for gonorrhoea. It seemed she had probably become reinfected since I'd first treated her.

It got worse. A couple of days later, Lizzy rang me in the middle of morning surgery.

'Sorry to interrupt, but it's a doctor on the phone from the GUM clinic. It's about Jean. Says it's urgent.'

I suddenly remembered Jean hadn't turned up for the scan I had arranged for her. Had the clinic discovered she had cancer after all?

'Hello, Rosemary.' It was Simon, an old friend from medical school. 'Jean, this patient of yours, her blood tests have come up positive. We've run the extra tests and it's confirmed – she's got syphilis.'

'She's what? How long do you reckon she's had it?'

'Difficult to say – probably at least five years. We need to get her into hospital for treatment.'

This wasn't going to be something I could arrange with Jean over the phone. And trying to get her into the surgery usually took a week of missed appointments. I decided the only option was to go round to her home.

Jean was delighted to see me. 'You should have rung,' she said. 'I'd have bought some nibbles, something bubbly and tidied up. What an honour. My lovely doctor is visiting me. Come in, come in, dear girl, out of the cold.'

Jean's flat was smelly, filthy and stuffed full of clutter, some of which looked valuable. Old books and papers spilled from every horizontal surface on to the threadbare carpet. Dusty ornaments, many of them broken, lay in piles on shelves and on the mantelpiece. In a display cupboard were framed yellowing photographs which I peered at as Jean swept some mess from a chair so that I could sit down.

I recognised a more youthful Jean in the photographs. She had been a stunner in her day, oozing class and wealth. Her serviceman husband had been matinée-idol handsome. They were pictured posing in beautiful clothes – she always in a hat and gloves – in front of imposing houses or grand cars. Here was evidence of a life which was a far cry from the sordid flat which was now her home. Jean offered me a cup of tea, which I politely declined. I'd seen the state of her kitchen, the sink full of dirty crockery, and it posed a serious health hazard.

'Your husband was a handsome chap,' I said, nodding towards the photos.

'Oh, Edward was drop-dead gorgeous,' she said. 'All the girls wanted him but I was the one he married. Delightful man, beautiful manners but as randy as a goat. He couldn't keep it in his pants, naughty boy, so I had to get used to sharing him. It didn't matter after a bit so I took lovers, too. I knew it was me that Edward adored. We had such a wonderful time in bed.'

I did some rapid mental calculations. The pictures I was looking at were just post war. So it was possible she'd had syphilis for fifty years . . .

'He died so young,' I said.

'Yes, tragic, he was just twenty-eight,' said Jean, 'but a long time ago now. We tried to have children but it didn't happen.'

Given their promiscuous lifestyle, Jean may have already had undiagnosed infections, not just with syphilis, which would have damaged her fallopian tubes and prevented her from getting pregnant, but I kept this thought to myself.

'I got a good pension from the Army,' continued Jean. 'That has kept the wolf from the door and I never felt like marrying again. What's the point, doctor? You just end up being a skivvy, washing their socks, cooking their meals, and I hate housekeeping and cleaning. We always had servants to do all that menial stuff when I was growing up. Men are handy in the bedroom and that's about it.

That's what I missed – the sex – so I did something about it. There are plenty of men out there who don't take much persuading. I've had a full life.'

I solemnly told Jean about the syphilis, trying to be as tactful as possible, and making loads of eye contact, while she watched me intently. As she leaned forward, I noticed that her pupils were very constricted.

When I finished, instead of exhibiting dismay or despair, Jean sat back, broke into a huge smile and clapped her hands in glee like a schoolgirl.

'Syphilis? What fun! Do you think this could be a record for someone of my age, doctor?' She wasn't remotely concerned. The only thing that upset her was when I said she had to stop having sex until we had sorted out her treatment.

Jean's face fell and I thought she might even cry. 'You can't be serious, doctor,' she said, aghast. 'I have sex every day with one of my gentleman friends. I'll miss it dreadfully and so will they. Please don't make me refrain from it.'

'It will just be for a bit, Jean,' I told her. 'But it's terribly important you refrain from sexual relations if we are going to make you well. Having that discharge can't have been much fun and you don't want that to come back, do you?'

Jean was looking daggers at me but then seemed to resign herself. 'OK, doctor. Just for a bit,' she said heavily. 'By the way, how long do you think I've had it?'

'It really is impossible to say – but many years. We need to get more tests done, but I think some of your memory problems may be due to the infection.'

Before the visit I'd gone back through her records. Normally a blood test for syphilis is done as part of the routine tests done in someone with dementia. Somehow Jean had never had it done.

In the absence of a positive blood test, syphilis is extremely difficult to diagnose. It is known as 'the great imitator' because its symptoms can be attributed to many other complaints.

After the first stage, when there is a sore which may not be noticeable and doesn't itch, the second stage is characterised by a rash which may be so mild it can go unnoticed. Then the disease can remain latent for years until the tertiary stage when it really starts to wreak havoc on the body – and that was the stage I suspected Jean had reached. The only good news, from a medical point of view, was that people with tertiary syphilis like Jean are no longer infectious, so she was unlikely to pass it on to anyone else, even if she did fall off the sexual wagon.

Many people today mistakenly think that syphilis is a disease of the past and, certainly, with the advent of penicillin in the last century, there was a huge dip in UK statistics.

However, in the early part of the twenty-first century, syphilis became slightly more common in the UK, with small outbreaks in Greater Manchester, London, Bristol and Brighton. In 2011, there were 2,915 new cases of syphilis diagnosed in the UK and, though the majority of these were men having sex with men, 291 were women, and 32 cases were in women over 45.

Up until the Second World War, some babies were born with the terrible disease of congenital syphilis, which they caught from their mothers. It resulted in blindness, deafness and brain damage.

Happily, this is seldom seen in Britain these days because every expectant mother gets a blood test for the infection. If it is discovered she is immediately treated – and cured – with antibiotics.

In Jean's case, blood tests and further investigations showed that she had indeed got tertiary syphilis and that her memory problems were probably not due to dementia at all but to neurosyphilis. In this the infection attacks the central nervous system and disrupts blood flow to the brain.

One of the classic signs of neurosyphilis are Argyll Robertson pupils. In a sufferer, the pupils constrict when they focus on near objects but do not constrict when exposed to bright light. I remembered how constricted her pupils had been when we talked in her flat. And, sure enough, when I checked, her pupils behaved like this and I wondered why the condition hadn't been picked up by her optician.

'Oh, I haven't had an eye test in years,' admitted Jean when I asked. 'It's a waste of time and money. I don't like wearing glasses – I'm too vain – and I only need them for reading. I can pick up a pair of reading specs in Tesco's and they suit me fine. I've got them in lots of different colours to match my outfits.'

Jean was treated with weekly penicillin injections. Every day when she was due for an appointment, one of the surgery staff would ring Jean to remind her to turn up. If time was getting on and we thought Jean had forgotten, Doreen would make one of her sons go round and collect her.

'You wouldn't believe it, doctor,' Doreen told me, eyes raised to heaven. 'She's even tried to proposition my boys.'

Irrepressible Jean still seems to regard the whole syphilis thing as a hoot and I wondered how seriously she had taken me when I tentatively suggested that she tone down her promiscuous lifestyle. I did toy with the idea of getting more heavy handed and referring her to a psychiatrist, with a view to having her 'sectioned' – compulsorily detained in a mental hospital. But I really didn't think her behaviour warranted that, and something in me didn't want all those self-righteous women from the church thinking they had got what they wanted.

Eventually, I think I got the 'safe sex' message across to Jean, encouraging her gentlemen friends to wear condoms, both to protect herself and them.

She thought the whole business was disgusting. 'Like paddling in wellington boots,' she said dismissively.

'Today's condoms are much better and thinner than they used to be,' I said, 'and you can get loads of different types and even different flavours.' To persuade her, the surgery gave her regular, free supplies. And there is evidence that she is using them because Jean is always singing the praises of flavoured condoms to anyone in the surgery who will listen.

'Fruits of the Forest is her favourite,' Lizzy told me. 'I always have to make sure she gets plenty of those or she kicks up a stink.'

'Well, as long as it does the trick.'

'Sounds like it,' said Lizzy.

'What do you mean?'

'Well, Jean has a rather loud voice and she always seems to find a male patient to sit next to when she comes in here. At first I thought she was talking to them about yoghurts but after the first complaint I looked more closely at the condom packaging . . .'

'So she's propositioning our male patients?'

'Yes she is, feisty old biddy. Well it's much warmer in the surgery for her; much more cosy than standing outside Tesco's or being frozen out by church wives.'

CHAPTER TEN

LEGS

Janet was what I'd call a 'bread-and-butter' patient – the sort of patient I see every day in the surgery who is not especially ill, but needs some assistance, of some sort, from their GP.

'Really sorry to bother you, Dr R, but I've had a bad tummy upset. Started off with being sick, and then diarrhoea. It's settling down now, but it's still not quite back to normal. And, as I work in the school kitchens, I can't go back till I get the all-clear from you. Sorry to bother you. I'm sure it'll only take a couple of days and I hate leaving the place short-staffed . . .'

'That's OK. I'd prefer to have just you off sick than half the school.'

'Exactly. I signed myself off for the first few days, but now it looks like I'm going to be off for more than a week, so I need a sick note from you.'

'No problem. And we'd better get a stool sample done, too, just be sure it's not salmonella or something like it.'

'Yes, thought you might say that.'

She grimaced as I handed her the sample pot, complete with a small spoon attached inside the lid. 'I'll leave it to you to work out how you collect the sample,' I grinned at her, 'and then leave it back at the front desk as soon as possible afterwards. Don't worry – the receptionists are used to little gifts of this kind.'

I reckon about a third of my consultations are made up of simple problems from 'bread and butter patients'. They come in with issues that can be solved in a relatively straightforward way and I then may not see the patient again for a couple of years, when they come in with something completely different. And then there are others, with more complex problems, who I see far more frequently.

Like Roger who was my next patient. My normal consulting room is at the top of a narrow flight of stairs, something that is often a problem for disabled patients. If a patient with a known walking problem is on my list for a surgery, the receptionists will arrange a swap with one of the other doctors into a consulting room on the ground floor. We didn't have Roger down as disabled on our list, but he made quite a meal of getting up the stairs and into my room, grimacing with every step and huffing and puffing when he got to the top.

Legs

He was forty-five and a painter by trade. He was of average height, nearing six feet, I reckoned, and he had a definite middle-aged paunch. Wearing tattered grey track-suit bottoms splattered with paint and a faded Adidas T-shirt, I guessed that he'd had to take some time out from doing a job locally to come into the surgery.

By the way that he walked in, grabbing his knees every so often, I wasn't surprised when he said, 'It's me knees doctor. Really painful all the time. It's worse when I walk.'

'Does it hurt in a particular place in your knee, or when you make particular movements?'

'Well, me left knee hurts more than me right. And it hurts all the time. I can hardly walk and, as you saw, stairs are a major problem.'

His answer wasn't quite what I was looking for, as it didn't really give me any of the further information I needed to start diagnosing the problem. I started on a different tack: 'Right. Could I possibly—'

Roger cut me short. His complaining wasn't over, 'Oh it really does hurt doctor. I'm a painter, you see, and I can't get up ladders, or do jobs properly. I can't do my job any more. I can't work.'

Gosh, I thought, this guy's laying it on thick. He's being very melodramatic. I had to be a bit more assertive to calm him down. 'Can I have a look at your knee? I can't do anything until I can see what's wrong with you.'

I managed to get him up on to the bed and I examined his knees. The left one was slightly inflamed and a bit stiff, but I couldn't find anything wrong with the right one.

I told Roger that he might have the beginnings of arthritis, but at this stage it was hard to tell. The best thing would be for him to take some anti-inflammatories. If the problem persisted then that ruled out a one-off knee injury and might indicate arthritis as a more likely cause.

'But what about my work? If I can't work, I can't pay the bills, and if I can't work 'cos of my knee I should get incapacity benefit.'

What Roger said was true. But it was way too soon for him to be talking about incapacity benefit. After all, this was the first time he'd come into the surgery with the problem. Even if the anti-inflammatories alone didn't sort the problem, I was sure there was nothing seriously wrong and some physiotherapy would soon have him walking normally again. Yes, it true that if you have a condition that means you are unable to work, you could be eligible for incapacity benefit but being unable to do the job you are currently doing is not enough – you need to be unable to work – at all. Roger's knee might have prevented him from his decorating job at the moment but, in my eyes, it didn't stop him from doing any kind of work whatsoever. Moreover, it's not me who decides whether he's fit for work or not, that's done by the Job Centre. They may ask the doctor for a report on the claimant's medical condition, but ultimately it's their decision. But now wasn't the time to get into an argument over benefits.

'Roger, it's early days. Take the anti-inflammatories and come back and see me in a week if nothing has improved.'

Roger begrudgingly hobbled out of my room and down the stairs, with similar vocal drama, as before.

My next patient put Roger's knees into perspective. Jack had been my patient ever since I'd become a doctor and moved to the area back in the late 1980s. When I first met him he was in his mid sixties. Looking much younger than his years, his face was unlined and there was not a grey hair to be seen. Dapper, trim and handsome, he had a slightly odd gait as he came into my room, but it took half an hour to get out of him why – he had two prosthetic legs below the knee. I never got many details (and he still won't tell me much to this day) but I eventually found out that he'd had the lower halves of his legs blown off in 1944 when his Spitfire crash-landed while defending south-east England from German bombers.

'It was a long time ago. At least I lived. Lots of my friends didn't. And, honestly, I've forgotten what it's like to have two normal legs. Just have to make the most of what's left of them. Hasn't stopped me having a great life. And rude good health.'

Very much the reluctant hero, Jack was very apologetic when he walked into the room. Even twenty years on from when I first met him, he still only had a few grey hairs and was as immaculately turned out as ever, and still looked fit and trim.

'Sorry to take up your time Rosemary, I'm sure you've got a lot of far more ill patients to see.'

Shrugging off his self-deprecation, I asked him what the problem was.

'I seem to be getting pain in my hips.' I'd suspected he could well have had pain in his hips for longer than he was letting on. The hip joints, a 'ball in a socket arrangement' are very susceptible to abnormal wear on the surface if the top of the main thigh bone, the 'ball', is not sitting absolutely centrally in the socket in the bone of the pelvis. Even slight unevenness when you walk can wear away an area of the protective cartilage covering the surface of the bone. While you could never see them, sixty years of walking on prosthetic lower legs almost certainly meant Jacks hips were not in a good way.

He didn't want to make a fuss. 'I was wondering if I could possibly get some physiotherapy to help. Shouldn't need much, just one or two sessions and some exercises to practise. I need to keep fit.'

If only some of my obese patients, who seemingly found it so difficult to do any meaningful exercise, could hear – and see – how someone as disabled as Jack still managed to be very active on a daily basis.

For a condition like his, physiotherapy certainly was an option. But if we did go down that route, one or two sessions was nowhere near enough. And, actually,

186

I wasn't sure that physiotherapy would help that much. The underlying problem was likely to be worn cartilage – not something physiotherapy can cure.

'Jack, I'll certainly refer you for some physio, but I think we should get your hips X-rayed as well. I think it would be helpful to see if there is any change in the structure of the joints. Whether the bones are rubbing together.'

'Oh no, no, no, there's no need for that. It's not that serious.'

'Are you sure? Only I don't want you suffering unnecessarily.'

'Let's try some physio first.'

I had to warn him he'd have to wait a few weeks. Inwardly that made me a bit cross. I felt that people like him – war heroes, no matter whether young or old, should have a bit of priority, but that wasn't the way the NHS seemed to work.

'That's OK. I'm sure there are others who need help more than me. And it's not stopping me doing my charity work – it's mainly desk based, though I do like to get out to meetings.'

'You are still working?'

'Of course, though I don't take any pay. Do it to help others, like me, and it also keeps my mind active – that's supposed to help delay the onset of dementia isn't it? And,' he added with a smile, 'it gets me out of the wife's way. We've just had our diamond anniversary and are still really happy. But I think that's because we give each other space. I don't think she could cope with me mooching around her all day long.'

What a lovely, sensible man.

A week to the day from when I first saw him, Roger the painter was back. The scene as he came up the stairs to my room was even more dramatic.

'This is no good at all, doctor. You shouldn't expect people to come upstairs to see you. You should have a room on the ground floor.'

'I know it's not ideal. Sorry. Come on in. How are your knees?'

'Bad, doctor, bad. Can hardly walk. Those pills you gave me have done nothing.'

'Let's have a look. Which one is worse?'

'The left. Can hardly bear to put any weight on it.'

I examined his knees and though there were many 'ooo's' and 'ouch's' coming from his mouth, I could find nothing wrong with them at all. The slight inflammation and stiffness I'd seen the last time appeared to have gone away.

'I don't think there's much wrong with them. Give the pills a bit longer.'

'Look, doctor, I've told you, those pills are doing nothing. I need proper treatment.'

'You've only tried them for a week. If you've got a small sprain, it's going to take longer than that to heal.'

'I tell you, doc, these knees are more than sprained. They are worn out.'

'Give it a bit longer,' I repeated and gently shooed him out of the door.

I was up in the kitchen a couple of weeks later when Naz walked in.

'I've just seen Roger, the bloke with the knee pain. Came to see me to get a sick note. Said he couldn't work because they were so painful.'

'Could you find anything wrong with them? Have I missed something?' I responded.

'Nope – couldn't find anything wrong at all. But he said he was in so much pain I felt I had to sign him off for a couple of weeks. And, being honest, my surgery was running so late I couldn't face having an argument with him.'

Next it was David's turn to deal with him. He brought it up at the next practice meeting.

'Roger, the bloke with the knees. Came to see me this morning. Wanted another sick note. He's doing the rounds of all of us, one by one. And none of us have found anything wrong. Who's going to take charge of this? Rosemary, you saw him first . . .'

I groaned.

'OK, then. Next person who sees him, tell him it's one doctor, one problem and to come back and see me. And you lot owe me,' I added, looking around the table. 'The next difficult patient goes to someone else.'

Roger was back in my room within a fortnight.

'You lot are all useless. No one's doing anything about the pain in my knees. Nothing has helped. I've seen the physio and she says she can't help either.'

That's probably because there's nothing wrong, I thought to myself.

'Let's get an X-ray done,' I suggested. 'That will show if there are any changes to the bones.'

'And if it's normal, what then?'

'Then your knees will get better.' That clearly wasn't the answer he was expecting.

My next patient was lovely Jack.

'So sorry to trouble you again, but I think you may have been right about having an X-ray done. I'm doing the exercises the physio suggested, but it feels like the bones are grating, especially on the right.'

I gave him the X-ray form and asked if he wanted any painkillers.

'No, I can manage with just an occasional paracetamol.' But he winced as he got up out of the chair.

Both X-ray results came back a week later. Roger's knees were completely normal, while Jack's hips were in a dreadful state. Both showed signs of advanced arthritis, and on the right, the space between the two bones, the ball of the femur and the socket of the pelvic bone, had nearly disappeared. That meant that the cartilage had worn away. It was a wonder he was still able to walk. The pain must have been awful.

I rang him up to save him the trouble of coming to the surgery.

'Jack, your right hip, I think it needs to be replaced. Can I arrange for you to see a specialist?'

'I was afraid you might say that. But it has been getting worse and the wife says she can hear it grating sometimes. So it's probably time I did something about it.'

I told him I'd get him seen as soon as possible. I rang Mike Wilkinson, my orthopaedic consultant friend, to see if there was some way Jack could jump the queue. He said he would see what he could do – he felt, like me, that war veterans should have some priority.

Most people are delighted when they hear that an X-ray they have had is normal. Roger wasn't one of them.

'What do you mean, my X-ray is normal? It can't be. What about all this pain? I need to see a specialist.'

Reluctantly, I agreed to refer him to Mike. Only this time, I thought, no phone calls. You can wait your turn.

A month later the phone rang. It was Lizzy, in reception.

'Roger, the knee bloke, is here. Wants to know why he hasn't got his hospital appointment yet. Is demanding to see you – and, of course, you haven't got any appointments. And I don't see why I should fit him in as an extra. It's not urgent.'

'Tell him we'll check with the hospital.'

'And he says that because he hasn't been seen he needs another sick note.'

I thought of Jack, still working hard at his desk, with his hip bones grinding together, and signed Roger off for another month. It's going to be that long before he's seen, I thought to myself.

He was back again, just as the month was up.

'I went to the hospital yesterday. Useless, bloody useless.'

'What happened?'

'Well, your mate, Mr Wilkinson, was away. So I saw his sidekick. Some Indian chap, who said there was nothing wrong with my knees that a bit of exercise wouldn't fix.'

I wasn't sure what to say. 'Well the X-rays were normal . . .'

'Bugger the X-rays. There's something wrong with my knees. I want to go to see someone who knows what they are talking about.'

'How about we wait until I get the letter back from the hospital?'

'Bugger that, too. I want to see someone who's going to tell me, properly, what's wrong with my knees. And meanwhile,' he added, glaring at me, 'I can't work, so I need another sick note.'

'Could you not do some office work at the building firm, if you can't paint?'

'No, it's painting or nothing for me. I'm not going to sit at a desk.'

Nothing wrong with sitting at a desk, I thought, as I sat at mine giving him yet another month off work.

The letter confirmed the orthopaedic specialist hadn't been able to find anything wrong with either of his knees. Which gave me a dilemma – why was he in such apparent pain, and was it justifiable to keep signing him off work?

He was back again as soon as his sick note ran out. Despite the dramas as he hobbled up the stairs to my room, I decided to take the bull by the horns.

'Roger, no one has been able to find anything wrong with your knees. I think you should try getting back to work.'

'By "no one" you mean the doctors here – well, none of you are experts, and neither is that bloke I saw at the hospital. I want to see someone who knows their stuff. I want a second opinion. And I've checked on my rights and, under the patient's charter, I'm entitled to see who I want.'

I hate patients quoting the patient's charter at me. I always try to do my best for my patients, but the NHS doesn't have a bottomless pit of money to cater for their every whim.

'Why don't I send you back to the same hospital and see if Mr Wilkinson can see you personally?'

'No way, he's a mate of yours. I want to go somewhere else, where I'll get a proper, independent opinion. I want to know what's wrong. I don't want to be told I just need to do a bit more exercise – especially when I can't, because of the pain. Bloody doctors. Have none of you ever had pain?'

I won't answer that one, I thought, thinking it was a shame he hadn't gone through the labour of childbirth. Twice.

I reluctantly agreed to refer him to see an orthopaedic surgeon at a different hospital. Again, the consultant could find nothing wrong when he examined Roger, but taking note that he was being asked for a second opinion, he arranged for an MRI scan. Unlike X-rays, which only show up changes in bony structure, an MRI can reveal changes in softer tissues, like ligaments and cartilage.

Soon after Roger saw the second consultant, Jack had his right hip replaced. I only knew when Enid, his wife, popped into the surgery to get a prescription for painkillers, a couple of days after he came home.

'Everything OK?' I enquired.

'Oh yes, he's fine. Though I think he maybe overdoing it a bit. He was given some exercises to do before he left hospital and no one said exactly how often he was to do them. He's at them at least once an hour. He's determined to be up and around, as normal, as soon as possible. Never complains about pain, though – I only know he's uncomfortable when he winces a bit, or I see him taking a painkiller. He never asks for help, even though he can't get his prosthesis on that side yet.'

How typical, I thought. 'Well, if you need anything, let me know. And tell him not to do the exercises so often if they cause pain.'

'I will, but I don't suppose he'll take much notice. There's a board meeting of the charity at the end of the month up in town, and he's determined to walk into the room, just as before – which means he's got to be able to get his prosthesis on. And you know what he's like – once he's set his mind to something . . .'

'Well, tell him to take care.'

Next day, Roger's MRI result came through. It was completely normal. That meant there really was no structural problem with his knee. I was chatting to Naz while we were waiting for the kettle to boil, when Doreen came in.

'You know Roger, that one with the knees who always hobbles in here with such drama? Well, I was fairly sure I saw him walking into the pub last week. Normally. No limp, nothing wrong with his walking at all. I didn't say anything, because I wasn't one hundred per cent sure it was him. But then, late yesterday afternoon, I saw him run across the road and into the bookies. And this time I got a really good view, and I'm sure it was him. Running fast I might add.'

'So there's nothing wrong with his knees.'

'Not from what I saw, no. Nothing wrong with them at all.'

'But I've only got your word for it. Has anyone else seen him out and about?'

'I'll ask the others and I'll get Lizzy to keep an eye out of the window upstairs, especially next time he's booked to come in. And maybe I'll have a little word with the lads who work at the bookies. And the butcher, you know, the one next door to the bookies, he knows exactly what's going on. And he owes us a favour – we're always patching him up when he's been a bit careless with his cleaver.'

Help, I thought, we're not just a doctors' surgery any more. We're turning into a detective agency.

Sure enough, all our 'spies' confirmed what Doreen had said. Outside the surgery, Roger could walk perfectly normally. And that, instead of working, he was occupying himself trying to make money at the bookies.

I hate conflict and I was dreading the next time he came in to the surgery demanding a sick note. But before he came in a letter arrived from the medical officer at the job centre. Roger had been called in for a medical examination, to assess his fitness to work, and he wanted a report from me beforehand. I answered the questions as accurately as I could, saying that nothing structurally wrong had been found with his knees and that no cause for his pain had been found.

I heard no more for a month. Then, one morning, I saw he was booked in to see me again. My heart sank. Please, I thought, not another demand for a sick note.

Yet again, there were hobbling scenes and cries of pain as he walked up the stairs. You chose the wrong profession, I thought. You should have been an actor. You wouldn't be walking like that if you'd had a last-minute tip off about the runners at the 3.15 at Doncaster. His face looked like thunder and he had barely got into the room before the tirade began.

'I've come to warn you, young lady,' he started. I didn't think that now was the time to tell him that I was older than he was. 'That I'm making a formal complaint about you. I'm going right to the top, the General Medical Council. But I've sent copies to your practice manager and also your bosses at the local health authority as well. You're a danger to patients. You shouldn't be allowed to practice.'

Despite my pulse racing, I kept calm. 'Come in and sit down.'

'Don't you try and sweet-talk me. You've done nothing to help me, and now you've lied to the job people.'

'Lied to the job people?'

'Oh yes. Lied through your pretty little teeth. Said nothing was wrong with my knees. How can you possibly say that when you have seen I'm in pain and can't walk properly?'

Tempting as it was to say it wasn't me who was the liar, but him, I didn't think it would get me anywhere. If anything it would only make matters worse. I decided to stick to the facts, and deliberately spoke quietly and firmly.

'I have a legal obligation to fill in forms asking for medical information as accurately as possible. I stated that no cause had been found for your pain.'

'Oh I know what you wrote. I've got a copy. You were deliberately negative. You said nothing about the problem

I have getting up to your room, did you? Said nothing about the pain I was in. I've checked the rules and you're supposed to be my advocate. That's what it says. You haven't been my advocate. And that's why I'm going to complain. You don't care about your patients, do you? All you care about is looking glam on the telly. Well, you're going to get your comeuppance, I tell you. The BBC won't want to know when they hear you're being investigated by the General Medical Council.'

I breathed a sigh of relief when he left the room. At least he hadn't asked for a sick note. But was he being serious about the complaint?

I found out soon enough – two days later in fact. Doreen came into my room at the end of morning surgery. She threw a three-page, typed letter on to my desk.

'Just look what that horrible man has gone and done.'

It was a copy of the complaint that had been sent to the Fitness to Practice panel at the General Medical Council (GMC).

I read it through.

'This is load of nonsense.'

'Yes, we know that, the bookies know that, the butcher knows that . . . but at the moment the GMC doesn't.'

'Oh gawd. I'll get on to my defence society.'

Like every doctor in the UK, I have full professional indemnity insurance. I've been told that every doctor has to expect at least one formal complaint during their career and most doctors have several.

Marie, the lawyer at the Medical Protection Society (MPS) was helpful and reassuring. She advised that I just had to stay calm, and go through the hoops of dealing with the complaint. Thank goodness she also warned me that it was also going to be time consuming and stressful. And it was, not just for me, but for my sons.

I knew I was innocent, but I was short fused at home. The boys learnt to give me a wide berth when I was working on my witness statement at home. And they kept their rooms tidier than usual. And for a while I didn't seem to have to find so many bits of sports kit, or music books, when I was trying to get ready for surgery in the morning. It seemed so unfair – I had done nothing wrong – and I kept thinking that some doctors would probably had been tougher and refused his end-less demands for sick notes. Was I a victim because I had been too soft? And was he deliberately gunning for me because I worked in the media? I'd always said to myself that if you put your head above the parapet, you have to expect to get shot at, and that as a celebrity of any sort you have to accept some criticism. But a complaint to the GMC for professional misconduct? That seemed grossly unfair.

Marie had warned me that, following on from the 'Shipman Business' a couple of years previously, the GMC had to be seen to be tough. They felt responsible that a GP in Lancashire had been able to kill some of his elderly patients and, as a result, benefit financially. It seemed that, for the time being at least, all GPs had been tarred, just a bit, with the same black brush.

'All complaints go through a set system,' she explained. There are several different panels; most get thrown out at the first or second one. It's only really serious complaints that end up with a formal hearing. I can't believe this one will go that far.'

'So I won't have to go and give evidence?'

'I doubt it. But, please understand, I can't be one hundred per cent sure. We'll just have to wait and see.'

As the date of the first panel hearing approached, I tried hard to stay calm. There's nothing more you can do, I thought to myself. I thought of all the hours of work I had put in getting all the paperwork ready. I really resented how long it had all taken.

Being honest, I expected Roger's complaint to be thrown out straight away. So it came as an almighty shock when Marie phoned and told me it had been referred up to the medical panel.

As before, she was reassuring.

'That's happening to all complaints at the moment, Rosemary. They are just really nervous after Shipman. The first panel is a lay panel. They're not doctors. I think they daren't do anything. Don't worry.'

Easier said than done. I lost my appetite, and found it hard to relax. And it wasn't just my home life that suffered. I found it difficult to practice good medicine – I started practicing defensive medicine instead. Ordering tests, and making referrals to specialists, 'just in case'. I had lost my self-confidence.

All the staff at the surgery knew what was going on, and were as supportive as possible. I had hoped none of the patients would notice anything different, but they were more observant than I gave them credit for. It was Jack who voiced their concerns. He had come to discuss his left hip.

'The right one went so well, I've decided I may as well get the other one done. I'm in my mid-eighties now – may as well stay as active as possible while I can. Goodness knows what's round the corner for me, or Enid. Time for us to live for the day. And, on that note, Rosemary, can I say something personal? Enid and I are worried about you. Actually, we're not the only ones. Seems the whole of Enid's bridge group is worried about you. We know you are one of life's copers, and you are bringing up those two lovely boys mainly on your own, but you've lost the glow in your cheeks. And you keep sending everyone for blood tests, and X-rays, and scans. And you've never done that before. Are you OK?'

What could I say without breaking patient confidentiality?

I was honest.

'Someone's made a complaint. To the GMC. I'm sure it will go away eventually but, yes, I'm finding it stressful.'

'You are a fabulous doctor. Would it help if I wrote to the GMC? This is ridiculous.'

'Thank you, but that's not quite the way it works. I just have to go through "the process" and it seems to be taking a long time. I'm trying not to think about it, but it's not easy.'

'We've all agreed you work too hard. You need to switch off. When did you last have a good game of tennis – or a holiday? Gosh, I'm sounding like you now – should we swap places?'

I laughed – for the first time in ages.

I didn't have to attend the hearing in person, as at this stage there was to be no input from the complainant or me. The panel of medics were merely reviewing the submitted written evidence. Though I'd been offered the morning off work on the day, I decided it was better to be distracted by patients than sit at home fretting. Even so, I was clockwatching all the time. I knew the panel was starting at 9am, but didn't know how many cases they had to plough through, or where mine was on the list. I just hoped I'd have some news by lunchtime.

The phone finally rang at 12.30.

'Rosemary?'

'Yes?'

'It's Marie. Good news. The complaint's been thrown out. Completely unfounded. You are completely in the clear. Not even the weeniest blemish on your character. Well done.'

'Thank you,' I breathed one of the largest sighs of relief ever.

Legs

The BBC never knew anything about it. I'd never seen any need to tell them but, yes, it had been a worry in the back of my mind. They wouldn't want any doubts about my professional competence. Was it a motive for the complaint? I'll never know.

As soon as the complaint had been thrown out, it was time to turn the tables. There was nothing I could do about all the time I had wasted dealing with the complaint, but I decided I couldn't possibly treat Roger again. After all, he had wrecked the doctor/patient relationship. The others all agreed. Doreen, in her typical forthright manner, expressed everyone's feelings very well: 'I don't want that lying son of a bitch in this surgery ever again.'

We had done our bit. It was time for another surgery to deal with his knees and pain. We threw him off our list.

CHAPTER ELEVEN

THE BUTTONED-UP BRIDE

Every so often a case comes along which knocks you sideways.

When I first saw Sashi at the surgery she had been married for two years and was very concerned about her inability to conceive. She was a healthy twenty-year-old, originally from Bangladesh but she and her family had immigrated to the UK from Sylhet, in the northern part of the country, four years previously. She had attended the local comprehensive school, spoke good English and, after she left school, had worked for a couple of years in a bank. Attractive, with huge brown eyes and a flawless café au lait complexion, she was dressed in western-style clothing, jeans and a T-shirt with a thick sweater, though she had modestly covered her hair with a hijab.

As we talked, I realised Sashi still held the very traditional views of a woman's role which persisted in her birth country. She certainly had an old-fashioned idea of how an ideal wife should behave. She had given up work completely when she married because she believed that a woman's place was in the home, serving her husband and making his life as comfortable as possible.

'I'm a bit bored actually,' she confessed. 'We live in a small flat, the housework and cooking does not take me long and without kids to keep me occupied, all I do is watch daytime TV.'

Latest estimates suggest there are now half a million Bangladeshis living in the UK. They are one of the largest immigrant groups in Britain and one of its youngest and fastest-growing communities. Marriage has a huge cultural significance and the average Bangladeshi wedding costs between £30–60,000 – a kind of downpayment for producing the next generation. Since her marriage, Sashi had been on the receiving end of relentless family and cultural pressure to produce a child, especially a son.

'I don't care what sex my child is,' Sashi told me, 'but everyone else seems to in the family, even my own mother. They have this really big thing about producing a son in my community.'

I made sympathetic noises. I was aware that in some hospitals, where there was a huge mix of diverse cultures, women were dissuaded, sometimes even not allowed, to find out the sex of the child they were carrying, for fear that they would terminate the pregnancy if they were expecting a girl.

Sashi sighed, 'Even if I do get pregnant, I will have to continue to have children until I get a son.' This seemed terribly unfair to me, especially as it is the father who determines the gender of a baby. If a woman becomes impregnated with a Y chromosome sperm, she has a boy; if it's an X, then she will have a daughter. She or her eggs have no say in it.

I wasn't sure that Sashi understood this when I explained it to her. She kept anxiously rubbing her hands as, eyes downcast, she confided that her family made her feel such a failure because no baby had arrived, in particular her husband's mother. 'I don't know what I am doing wrong,' she said. 'I try to be a good wife to Aarif. We love each other very much and we are very affectionate.' She blushed and I thought I had got the picture. No problems in bed, then. But she seemed to be taking all the blame on to herself.

'Sashi – it takes two to make a baby. Not just you – but your husband as well. It might not be your fault.'

The look of disbelief she gave me revealed that this had simply not occurred to her.

She and Aarif had barely known each other before their wedding and she explained that theirs had been an arranged marriage. Catching my look of apprehension, she was quick to disabuse me of any prejudice.

'I was happy for it to be arranged. My family knew Aarif and his family and they chose very wisely for me. Aarif and I are very happy and he is a very handsome man, just two years older than me. He's kind and gentle and he makes me a laugh a lot, but he does want to become a father and I feel I am failing him.

'He never makes me feel guilty – he loves me – but he has a large family and they have made many unkind comments. I think they want him to cast me aside.' Sashi's eyes filled with tears and I pushed the tissues I always keep on my desk towards her.

Sashi said her most venomous critic was Aarif's widowed mother, who lived with his older sister Farhana and her husband a few doors away in the same street.

'Farhana's only a year older than me but she already has three children and one of them's a son,' said Sashi. 'I don't know why my mother-in-law thinks it's so important for me to have a baby; she's got plenty of grandchildren to dote on already. I guess it's the way she was brought up herself. Whenever she visits our house she always brings her knitting. And guess what she's making? Blue baby clothes. Talk about pressure – she never lets up.'

Sashi's tears were flowing freely and I waited until she had composed herself before I questioned her further. Then I asked the usual questions one asks when exploring possible infertility.

'Do you have regular monthly periods, or are they sometimes a bit erratic?'

'They are very regular – I can predict when I'm going to bleed, almost to the hour. And now, of course, I dread it – I know it means I'm not pregnant.'

'What about pain – are your periods painful, or do you get any pain in your pelvis during sex?' Very painful periods can be a symptom of endometriosis, or a pelvic infection, which can be linked with fertility problems.

'No – I have slight twinges when my period starts, but nothing too bad. And no pain inside during lovemaking.'

I moved on to sexual history to look for other clues. Had Sashi or Aarif ever being diagnosed with a sexually transmitted infection? Had she been pregnant before, or had her husband fathered previous children?

Sashi could not have looked more mortified if I had asked if she turned tricks on street corners. She was so affronted I feared she might walk out. With barely restrained temper, she said, 'Aarif and I were both virgins when we got married. We did not even touch each other before our wedding day, although we both wanted to. Of course, we have never had any children before we met – we are both pure. How could you suggest such a thing?'

Her clothing had misled me – she was much more traditional in her beliefs than I had realised. I apologised for offending her and moved on to the tricky question about the frequency and timing of sex. Though I was wary of upsetting her again, it was my duty to probe this sensitive area. Many couples do not realise that there only a few days a month when a woman can get pregnant and that is around the time she ovulates, or releases an egg from one of her ovaries. The female egg lives only for twenty-four hours maximum after ovulation, while a man's sperm can survive for up to five days in the female genital tract waiting to ambush it. So for a woman like Sashi with a standard twenty-eight-day cycle, the best time to have sex if she wanted to get pregnant would be between day nine and fourteen of her monthly cycle. Again, she looked rather puzzled but I said I would run some tests to see if her body was functioning properly.

Carrying out hormone tests to discover if a woman's ovaries are working normally is not entirely straightforward. One has to be done between days two and four of her cycle (i.e. during her period). This checks for levels of Follicle Stimulating Hormone (FSH) and Luteinising Hormone (LH) which, when produced in the right amounts, ensure normal ovulation. Another test assesses progesterone levels, a hormone that creates a fertile environment for conception. This one has to be done a week after the calculated ovulation date, usually around day twenty-one.

At the same time as arranging these, I also asked if we could arrange to carry out a semen analysis on Aarif. Sashi was dismayed. 'But why doctor? It's me who can't get pregnant.' I obviously hadn't got through to her, so I patiently reiterated my 'it takes two to make a baby' speech. I also explained that sometimes a man can have a low sperm count which makes it difficult for his partner to conceive and it was just as important to check this out as to do tests on her. I was beginning to wonder how naive this married woman really was. Even then I failed to grasp the depths of her innocence.

I spoke to my colleague Naz about Sashi's case. Naz was born in Pakistan but came to Britain in her early childhood.

'I know you didn't come from Bangladesh like Sashi, but do you have any ideas? I don't much like this arranged marriage idea but then I'm bringing western prejudice to the subject.'

'Oh, I had an arranged marriage,' said Naz and laughed when she saw my horrified look. 'It's worked for me, Rosemary. But then I arranged it myself.'

'How come?'

'I'd had my eye on Tariq for some time,' said Naz. 'I told my parents that if they did not arrange for me to marry him, I would run away from home and have a baby with a white Roman Catholic. Fortunately, they could see how hot Tariq and I were for each other and were so frightened that I would leap on him and disrupt his medical studies by having his child that they gave in without much of a fight. They liked him anyway, so that helped.'

Naz thought for a bit. 'It might be more to do with Sashi's upbringing than her ethnic background,' she said. 'Some mums, irrespective of race, are so keen to keep their daughters virgins that they don't tell them anything and stonewall all their questions about sex.'

'But surely they talk with their friends . . .'

'She's a shy girl, right?'

'Yes, she is.'

'Well she probably hangs around with other shy girls and shuts her ears to anything she believes is gratuitous crudeness. She's probably been over-protected. And since she was sixteen when she arrived here, she almost certainly missed any sex education – it's done when kids are much younger than that.'

'Yet she says she enjoys having sex with her husband . . .'

'It's a puzzle, Rosemary, and I'm sorry but I have no idea either.'

Sashi's test results revealed that everything was fine, which was what I had expected. That led me to think that the problem probably lay with her husband.

When I first started work as a GP, most of the cases of infertility I saw were due either to ovulation problems, blocked fallopian tubes, or they had no identified cause. But over the past twenty years, the pattern has changed and, though stories in the press often concentrate on the female side of things, in at least half the cases there appears to be a problem with sperm production. Sperm counts have been falling dramatically in Britain over the past half-century and many reasons have been cited. In America, statistics reveal that in the past fifty years, the sperm count of the average American male has dropped from 120 million sperm per millilitre of semen to just over 50 million, and in Britain the fall is similar.

There are many biological and environmental factors in our modern age that can lead to male infertility and damaged sperm, such as oestrogen-like chemicals in the water supply, thought to originate from pesticides and also from hormone-based contraceptives taken by women.

Smoking can certainly affect the sperm count, too, and drinking too much alcohol can not only lower sperm counts but damage developing sperm. Sperm production can be slowed down by keeping the scrotum too hot and, though wearing tight-fitting underwear is often mentioned, in reality this is probably only of importance in men who have a borderline low sperm count.

Sport is usually beneficial but certain types of exercise can adversely affect sperm and one of the worst culprits is cycling. Mountain bikers have registered less than half the sperm count and sperm movement of non-cyclists because of the impounding damage to the scrotum and testes.

Taking anabolic steroids to increase performance in sports, such as weight lifting, and using banned substances, such as cocaine, marijuana and heroin, can reduce sperm production by up to half and cause permanent infertility in a man.

Some illnesses such as cystic fibrosis can cause male infertility but a more common cause is varicocele – an enlarged or twisted vein in the cord that connects to the testicle. Varicoceles are found in twenty to fifty per cent of all men and in twenty-five to forty per cent of infertile men. There is no conclusive reason why, but theories put forward include obstructing the passage of sperm, raising the temperature or producing higher levels of nitric oxide, a substance that will damage them.

Sashi's husband Aarif was happy to cooperate in the tests to see if he was producing adequate sperm. He seemed a very kind, gentle and caring man, and he held his wife's hand as we talked together.

'I've had a hard time convincing Sashi that I don't mind doing this,' he told me. 'I'll try anything, doctor. This whole business is making my wife so unhappy. I am longing to be a father but I don't want to make Sashi miserable. I've told her to take no notice of my family – I know they are being unfair to her – but she is a very sensitive person and has become very distressed.'

I asked Aarif what he did for a living, wondering if there might be infertility clues there.

'I am an electrician,' he said. I did not think that would prevent him from becoming a father and looked for other obvious reasons. However, Aarif did not cycle, smoke or take drugs, nor did he drink alcohol. When I received his results it transpired that his sperm count was normal, too.

'Sashi is getting so worried about this. It would really help if we could see a specialist. Is that possible?' he asked me.

I wasn't sure it was justified, at least not quite so soon. I told Sashi I'd discuss their case at our next referrals meeting. This was a recent addition to our meeting schedule, to check whether the referrals we were making to hospital clinics were appropriate. Though it was introduced by our Primary Care Trust as a means of potentially saving money, we all found it useful. As a GP, it's easy to get into bad habits and send a patient off to see a hospital specialist when they could be dealt with just as effectively by a colleague with different skills within the surgery. It's also a means of checking that all the relevant tests have been done before a patient is referred. 'She's so young and they've only been married for two years – is it reasonable for me to wait a bit and let nature take its course?'

It was agreed at the meeting that the next step should be to arrange a scan to see if anything was amiss in her pelvis, and to try and persuade them to 'keep trying' in the meantime. As Sashi didn't have any gynaecological symptoms, was only twenty-two and had had sex with only one man, I didn't consider a vaginal examination necessary. In retrospect, this was a big mistake and could have avoided a great deal of heartache, but it's easy to be wise in hindsight. I could have carried it out then and there, but there just didn't seem to be any reason to put her through it.

I explained that the scan would be done via Sashi's vagina, which gives a far better image than the old-fashioned way of scanning through the abdominal wall. With that method, women were advised to have full bladders before a scan to improve image quality and often had problems maintaining control.

I told Sashi that, as she was a married woman who enjoyed regular sex, the vaginal scan shouldn't hurt. 'As long as you relax it shouldn't even be uncomfortable,' I assured her.

But when Sashi returned three weeks later on the day after her scan, she was very angry. She stomped into my consulting room, brown eyes blazing, none of the passive female about her at all this time. 'Why didn't you warn me that examination was going to hurt so much and that I would bleed afterwards?' she accused furiously before she had even sat down.

'It shouldn't have done,' I said. What on earth had gone on? I thought to myself. A scan shouldn't hurt or make her bleed. 'Let me read the scan report and I will try to find out why.' She waited, barely mollified, while I read, hoping it would throw more light on the subject. It did not. The ultrasonographer had not been able to get a decent view of Sashi's pelvis because the patient had found the procedure too painful.

And now Sashi was bleeding. Something wasn't right. This time I had to get her on the couch to examine her internally.

The moment I tried to insert a speculum into her vagina Sashi tensed up so much it became impossible to continue. It made me wonder if sex had been hurting her, too. 'Does intercourse hurt?' I asked her.

'Sex is nothing like this,' she replied. 'My husband doesn't go in the place where you tried to put that horrible thing.'

I wasn't so much shocked as incredulous. Did that mean she was having anal sex? And, if so, why? Was it through ignorance or her husband's preference? I had no idea.

I felt it was time that Sashi, still lying on the couch, recovering from the abandoned internal examination, had a basic anatomy lesson. 'You can't get pregnant if you are having sex via your back passage,' I told her gently. 'You need to have sex here,' and I pointed to her vagina, 'not here,' I continued, indicating her anus.

She looked at me as if I was crazy. 'But Aarif doesn't go anywhere near there,' she practically screeched at me. 'And he doesn't go in that other place where I have my monthly bleeds. That's private, for me alone.'

'Where does he go, then?' I asked weakly, thinking I had exhausted all reasonable options. Sashi put her hand on her stomach and pointed to her navel. 'Here,' she said. 'This is where babies come from. My mother told me it is the source of all their nourishment.'

Surely she wasn't being serious. Not trusting myself to speak, I inspected her belly button. It looked red and sore, as if it had been rubbed very vigorously. Was she trying to tell me that she had been having sex in her navel? Indeed, she was.

It does seem unbelievable, I know, that in the twenty-first century, when there is so much information about sex on TV and in newspapers and magazines, that this young couple could be so ignorant about it but, I suppose, Sashi and Aarif had both had very sheltered upbringings and no one had ever informed them about the basic facts of life. All Sashi had been taught was that it was a woman's duty to bear children. It seemed she had been told how a baby grew inside the womb, but no one had ever told her how it got there in the first place. Even now, as I spelt it out to

217

her, I wasn't sure she was grasping it. She seemed disgusted and horrified.

Luckily, because my practice is in south London, which has a very diverse multicultural population, I was able to arrange for Sashi to see a counsellor from Bangladesh.

I had wondered whether she would change doctors when the facts of life were explained to her because she would be too embarrassed to see me again, but she didn't. When I saw her a few months later, it was to confirm her first pregnancy. Neither of us mentioned her navel, I just focused on her impending motherhood.

Sashi got a son first time around and there were no complications surrounding his birth. He had plenty of blue knitted baby clothes waiting for him and I'm sure Sashi's relationship with her mother-in-law improved immensely. I never discovered whether Sashi actually enjoyed vaginal sex, or whether it was merely a means for her to have a baby. There are some questions which I reckon are best left unasked.

CHAPTER TWELVE

THE POWER OF THE PRESS

It was a bright morning in June 2006. I was on visiting duty and, for once, there weren't many listed in the book.

Lizzy suggested I see little Fleur first.

'Her mother sounded really anxious when she phoned. Asked if you could go round as soon as possible. That's unusual for her. I think she's worried it's meningitis, though from what she said, the symptoms don't sound quite right. Something about a temperature and really red eyes.'

'Did she say anything about a rash?' I enquired.

'Yes – and that's what makes me think it's not meningitis. She said she'd done the glass test and it blanched – which means it's not the meningitis rash?'

'Correct. Well done. The septicaemia rash, that can occur with meningitis, is caused by bruising under the skin and, unlike other rashes, it stays the same when you press on it with a glass. Fleur's probably just got a minor viral infection but, even so, there are no other urgent visits, so I'll do that one first.'

I sped off to a quiet, tree-lined street of late Victorian semi-detached houses in a desirable part of south-east London. I eventually found a place to park my little hatchback among the Mercedes estates and premium 4x4s, and began to look for number sixty-five. It was a fine day in the summer, the leaves were out on the immaculate hedges adorning people's front gardens and the sun was highlighting the various tasteful colours of the front doors. It was certainly one of the more pleasant approaches to a home visit.

Number sixty-five's front door was a delicate shade of pale green that matched what looked like original Victorian tiles that lined the sides of the porch, with a replica Victorian glass lantern adorning the ceiling. I looked for the bell, but realised this was not the type of house that would play a tune on the press of a button. Instead, I used the ornate brass knocker. I was greeted at the front door by Julia, Fleur's mother, a lady in her mid-thirties, with a bohemian air about her, wearing a long, linen skirt and a loose linen T-shirt, with a large coloured stone necklace. I was led to the front room. The large bay window had heavy, patterned curtains drawn across, while the sofas were adorned with throws. Little trinkets clearly collected from all over the world adorned shelving either side of the fireplace, while on the coffee table were two stained mugs, a packet of organic biscuits, several interior design magazines and a copy of both the *Daily Mail* and the *Guardian*.

Little Fleur looked really unwell, a far cry from the lively five-year-old who had come into my surgery only a couple of weeks previously with a sprained ankle – acquired while jumping a little too vigorously on the trampoline in her back garden. She lay curled up in a ball on the sofa, under her pink flowery duvet, her little legs tucked under her tummy.

'I'm so sorry to call you out,' Julia started apologetically. 'I know it makes extra work for you but I don't think she could sit in the waiting room. She just wants to lie down all the time. I didn't even dare leave her upstairs on her own. I had to bring her down here where I could keep an eye on her while I got on with the chores. And I can get on with my work if I sit beside her.'

Fleur was not remotely interested in anything going on around her. Her eyes were red and watery, and periodically she had bouts of harsh, dry coughing. Her head and neck were smothered in a blotchy red rash and when I laid a hand gently on her forehead, I could tell that she had a raging fever. I checked inside her ears and found both the canals and her ear drums to be red and inflamed. I had a good idea what was wrong with her, but needed one more piece of evidence to complete the diagnostic jigsaw puzzle. I gently asked her to open her mouth, as wide as possible, so I could examine the inside of her cheeks. I found what I was looking for – small white spots.

I turned to her mother and I could see Julia's face was etched with worry.

'What is it? What's wrong with her? Is it meningitis?'

'No, it's not meningitis. Not quite as bad – but nearly. It's measles.' I was being very serious. Measles is not the 'mild viral illness' I had been expecting.

'Measles? How can it be? No one gets measles anymore.'

'It's true that until recently cases of measles have been fairly rare, but in the last few months the number has been going up again, dramatically, especially here in south London.'

'Why?'

I decided in this case not to answer Julia's question directly, but to answer her inquiry with a question of my own. It was one of those when I was pretty sure of the answer before I'd even asked the question.

'Julia, did Fleur have all her MMR vaccinations?'

She looked defiant, 'No. She's had a single jab against rubella, because I know that if she had German measles when she's older and happened to be pregnant, then the baby could be affected. So girls need to be protected against that. And I was thinking about getting her a single jab against mumps. But the measles jab just seems too risky. And not necessary, because I thought measles had gone away. Are you sure it's that?'

'Yes, I'm fairly sure, but I need to take some swabs to be certain. I'll get the result back as quickly as I can.'

'But, in the meantime, you'll give her some strong antibiotics?'

'No, there's no point. Measles is caused by a virus. Antibiotics only help fight infections caused by bacteria. They won't be any help with this.'

'What? So what treatment are you going to give her?'

'There isn't any treatment for measles, other than paracetamol and ibuprofen to help reduce her raging fever and ease her aches and pain.'

'You're telling me there's no treatment for measles? That can't be right in this day and age. There must be something.'

'No, I'm afraid there is nothing. If there was anything, of course I would prescribe it straight away, but there isn't.'

'Why wasn't I told this before?'

Now was not the time to tell her that, actually, she had been told this before. I remembered the difficult conversation I'd had with her when she'd refused to let Fleur have the MMR. And, to be fair, she wasn't alone. There were lots of mothers in the area who had acted in exactly the same way because they were convinced the vaccine was both dangerous and unnecessary.

It all started with a paper that was published in *The Lancet* in 1998, written by Dr Andrew Wakefield and some of his colleagues at the Royal Free Hospital in London. It supposedly presented evidence that the MMR vaccine was linked to the development of autistic spectrum disorders in children. Wakefield suggested that, in the interests of safety, children should not be given the MMR vaccine and if parents wanted to give them protection, they should be given the single components of the vaccine – measles, mumps and rubella – separately. The real reason for this suggestion – that he had a vested interest in undermining public confidence in the MMR – would only become apparent many years later.

At the time, Wakefield's original paper garnered only limited press attention. The fact that it garnered any mainstream press attention at all was surprising. Many hundreds of drug research papers are published every year and only a very few ever make it into the mainstream press. More surprisingly, it made it into the mainstream press despite it being terrible research.

Only twelve children were studied. In the world of medical research, a study of twelve patients is tiny and almost laughable. In order to have meaningful results in any drugs trial, you need to have enough patients to be confident that what you are studying (the effect of the drug/vaccine) is what is causing the effect you are actually observing (in Wakefield's case, the onset of autistic spectrum disorders). You have to be sure that it's not some other factor (what they're eating, what other conditions they might have, their genetic make-up; it could be anything) that's causing what you're observing, or that it's not just coincidence that the particular patients you're observing develop a condition after taking a drug/vaccine. Just because one thing occurs after another, it doesn't mean that the first thing *caused* the second.

To this end, a typical piece of drugs research today will have hundreds, if not thousands, of patients participating. Drug companies and the bodies that license drugs recognise that you cannot have meaningful results in your research unless you have a large body of patients. There were other (arguably bigger) problems with Wakefield's research, such as the fact that some of his treatment of the child patients in the study was unethical and also that he falsified his results. But at the time we weren't aware of them.

Though his initial paper didn't get much attention, Wakefield didn't get off his hobby horse. In 2001 and 2002 he published further papers in minor journals. Some of the papers contained no new evidence. Others contained 'evidence' (later found to be utterly meaningless) that he had found the measles virus in tissue samples taken from children who had autistic spectrum disorders. Crucially, Wakefield this time went further than his initial claim that it might be prudent to suspend the MMR vaccine pending further research. This time he claimed that the NHS MMR vaccination programme was unsafe.

Suddenly the press machine went into overdrive. More and more articles appeared, most of them coming out in support of parents who claimed their children's autism was caused by the MMR. Most of the articles were being written by general journalists, who hadn't the scientific background to see the flaws in the research. The fact that the symptoms of autism – which is mainly a disorder of social communication – start in the second year of life and so, inevitably, would start after the MMR is given at age thirteen months was ignored. For a journalist, the story had real sales potential – anecdotes from distraught parents blaming a lazy government for giving their child a vaccine that had left them autistic.

Between 1998 and 2002, I worked for the *Daily Mail* as their resident GP. I had a weekly column, most of which was answering questions from readers. Most of my columns didn't bear much relation to the headlines of the day and I was very rarely called upon to get involved in the 'news' section of the paper. When MMR hit the papers, though, all that changed. The two sides of my professional life – working as a doctor and working as a journalist – collided head on.

As the story grew, I was approached from all sides. The journalists on the *Daily Mail* were calling me to get advice or a comment for the latest news article. Many of them were left disappointed when I refused to endorse the research, endorse parents' claims of malpractice or condemn the MMR vaccine.

For the *Daily Mail*, the terrible research that under-pinned the link to autism was an inconvenient truth that got in the way of a good story. I refused to allow my name to be added to the media circus calling for the end of MMR. I stuck to the line being given out by the official committee on vaccination and immunisation. I was well aware that the committee was staffed by extremely experienced doctors and scientists working in the field of immunisation and I knew that Wakefield's claims had been examined very carefully, especially in light of all the media attention. The committee checked all research done on the vaccine – on hundreds of thousands of patients worldwide, and reiterated its excellent safety record, and that no link with autism had been found, other than in the twelve patients studied by Wakefield.

At the same time, I was faced with a dilemma. My salary from the *Daily Mail* was helping to pay my hefty mortgage, and I knew every time I refused to toe the line my job was made less secure. I had previously been fired overnight from the *Sun* because my face didn't fit when the editor changed, so I knew how brutal the media industry can be.

But I was also well aware of how potentially damaging this story was. At the time it started, measles had become a rare condition. But if vaccination rates fell, then the disease could rear its ugly head again, and I still had memories from my own childhood of just how frightening it could be.

My younger sister Margaret caught measles in 1967, when she was three, and I was eleven. It was a bad year for measles in the UK. There were over 460,000 recorded cases, and 90 deaths, most of them young children. Margaret was delirious for three days and, on the instructions of our family doctor, someone had to sit with her, day and night, to be sure she didn't slip into a coma. Along with my older sister, I took my turn at Margaret's bedside, with instructions to rouse her every hour. In retrospect, she almost certainly had mild encephalitis, or inflammation of the brain, a well-known complication of measles.

Margaret was one of the lucky ones. Even though she was severely ill, she came through it unscathed and made a full recovery.

I had been coming to the end of a surgery one morning in the spring of 2002 when Fiona, the practice nurse, buzzed me through. She sounded exasperated.

'I've got another one with me who's refusing the MMR. Whatever I say I can't persuade her, but she says she'll come and have a chat with you. Can I fit her in with you as an extra?'

My heart sank, but I knew I couldn't say no.

'Of course, who is it?'

'Julia. Fleur's mother.'

That surprised me. Julia had always come across as an eminently sensible mother. And well informed. Too well informed now, I thought. How had she managed to be sucked into the scaremongering?

'Can you ask her to wait while I see my last couple of booked patients? I'll be able to spend more time with her if I see her at the end.'

The Power of the Press

Julia came in, with thirteen-month-old Fleur bouncing on her left hip.

'This whole business is awful, I just don't know what to believe,' she started. 'Fleur is so healthy, I just don't want to give her anything that could damage her.'

I nodded sympathetically. 'I understand your anxiety, but can I just go through the facts with you?'

I explained how Wakefield's research had only been done on twelve children, and yet the vaccine had been used with no problems on hundreds of thousands of children worldwide. I also explained how symptoms of autism often appear in the second year of life and as the cause wasn't known, parents wanted something, anything, to blame.

'But that's just it,' replied Julia. 'The cause of autism isn't known. What if it is the MMR? I just can't bear the thought of giving it to Fleur and possibly making her autistic. Every day I keep reading in the paper how dangerous this vaccine can be.'

I was honest with her. 'Julia, I've had odd moments of doubt in the back of my mind, too. I've had conversations like this several times each week and occasionally I have thought, "What if it isn't quite as safe as I think? Should I be pushing this vaccine – like I am, right now, with you?" Then I look again at the research data and until someone else comes up with more data to support Wakefield's claims, I still believe the vaccine should be given. Children need to be protected from these diseases.'

'I understand why rubella is dangerous for girls, but measles and mumps? Neither are that serious and, anyway, they are not around anymore.'

'They are only "not around" because children have been vaccinated. Odd cases do still occur in susceptible children and both diseases can be nasty. Mumps can cause inflammation of the ovaries and testes, and cause infertility, while measles can cause deafness and brain damage. Occasionally it kills.'

I recalled the tale of sitting with my younger sister.

'But that was back in the mid sixties. That's ages ago. There are treatments for diseases now.'

'No there aren't. All these illnesses are caused by viruses and antibiotics are of no help at all. Even now, in the twenty-first century, there is no treatment for either of them.'

'Have your boys had the vaccine?'

'Yes, both of them. Two doses each.'

'That's a better argument for the vaccine than anything else you've said. I know how important those boys are to you. You wouldn't do anything to harm them.'

She wasn't the first patient who had said that. Up until that moment, I was being labelled as just another doctor joining in the conspiracy of silence over a potentially damaging vaccine. But when I spoke as a mother – well, that was way more important than my medical training!

'I'm still not sure. It's the measles component I'm really scared about. But I'll have a think about giving her the single rubella vaccine. I know girls need to be protected against German measles.'

There never was, and never has been, any evidence that giving the jabs against measles, mumps and rubella separately is any safer than giving them all together. It seems that part of the reason Wakefield came up with the idea was because he had a financial interest in undermining confidence in the MMR vaccine, hoping to sell diagnostic kits, and, eventually, his own replacement vaccine. Many parents, doing what they must have thought was the best for their children, took them to private clinics to have single vaccines. The single jabs were unlicensed, which meant they had not been through the rigorous safety checks demanded by law for licensed products. Yet many of my patients chose this option – which I thought was very unfair on their children. Not only were the children being given jabs of potentially dubious provenance and quality, but to be fully immunised a child had to have six separate jabs, several weeks apart, rather than just two. Of course, what actually happened was that most children had one or two jabs – hardly any had all six, and many, like Fleur, remained susceptible to measles, and often to mumps or rubella as well.

The story was at its peak in early 2002, with politicians being called on to say whether their children had been vaccinated using MMR. Tony Blair (rightly, in my view) refused to comment on whether Leo was given the MMR (though in 2010 Cherie, in her autobiography, confirmed that he had). I was getting regular calls from the *Daily Mail* and was regularly refusing to contribute to their sensationalism and, at the same time, directly contradicting their stories when I appeared on *BBC Breakfast*. Whenever I went on air to comment on the MMR story I did my level best to stress that extensive good research on the vaccine had proved that it was safe.

In the MMR war, I was fighting a battle on two fronts. I was fighting a battle against the *Daily Mail* and their insatiable urge for sensationalist stories and, at the same time, I was fighting a daily battle against falling vaccination rates in my surgery, trying to convince parents to have their children vaccinated.

Between 1996 and 2002, MMR immunisation rates dropped from ninety-two to eighty-four per cent. In 2003, in some parts of London, including the area where I worked, that rate was as low as sixty-one per cent. That meant that sooner or later there was bound to be an outbreak of measles.

Low vaccination rates have a double effect. When vaccination rates are high, above ninety per cent, the minority who aren't vaccinated are effectively protected from the disease by the majority who are. Measles is an infectious disease, so you generally catch it from someone else who has it. If everyone else is immunised against measles, it's quite hard to catch it even if you're not immunised. When vaccination rates fall, this effect, which is known as Herd Immunity, disappears. Having herd immunity disrupts the chain of infection. This explains the dramatic rise in the number of measles, mumps and rubella outbreaks, despite on paper the vaccination rate only falling eight per cent between 1996 and 2002. In 1996 there were fifty-six confirmed cases of measles in the UK, in 2006 there were 449 from January to June alone. Measles, being the 'nastiest' of the three diseases, received the most attention, but for mumps the story is even worse. There were thirty-seven times more cases of mumps in 2006 than there were in 1998.

In the summer of 2006 we had already had two cases of measles in the practice and there were several others in the area. I rang the Health Protection Agency from Julia's house, to organize the swabs that were needed to confirm the diagnosis. Meanwhile, I advised Julia to give Fleur regular paracetamol to try and control her temperature, and also encourage her to drink as much as possible. I recommended giving her ice lollies to suck if she found swallowing too painful.

'And call me if anything changes,' I added. 'For instance, if she starts vomiting or appears more drowsy or confused.'

The swab results came through very fast, and I phoned Julia to tell her Fleur definitely had measles.

'I'm so glad you've called,' she sounded anxious and was speaking fast. 'She's worse than yesterday. I can't get her fever down at all, she's barely drinking, and she wants to lie in the dark. She says the lights hurt her eyes.'

Alarm bells started ringing in my head. Dislike of bright light – photophobia – can be a sign of meningitis, which can be a complication of measles. Officially I wasn't doing visits that day, but as I'd seen her yesterday I would be the best person to judge if her condition really had deteriorated. I said I'd call round at the end of surgery.

I hit the knocker, but there was no reply. I waited a few minutes, then hit it again. Eventually Julia came rushing to the door, looking dishevelled.

'So sorry, Fleur's just been sick. It's gone everywhere . . .'

Good thing I'm wearing a cotton dress that I can throw into the machine then, I thought to myself.

In fact, there wasn't much mess because Fleur hadn't been eating and had hardly been drinking either. She didn't want to move or open her eyes.

'Everything hurts, especially my head and eyes.'

'Can you open them for me just a bit?'

'No, just leave me alone.'

'Come on, Fleur,' Julia encouraged her, 'just let Dr Leonard have a look, so she knows how to make you better.'

I caught a glimpse of Fleur's red, blood-shot eyes as she briefly opened them.

'Fleur, I'm just going to gently move your neck, is that OK?' I asked her

She didn't reply.

As I tried to flex her neck forwards, she burst into tears

of real pain. Her skin was hot and clammy, and her mouth was bone dry.

'Julia, I think she needs to go to hospital – she's dehydrated,' I explained. 'And I'm concerned now that has got meningitis.'

'But yesterday you said she hadn't? You said the rash wasn't right for that.'

'Not meningococcal meningitis, which is the one everyone knows about. I think the lining of her brain – the meninges – may be inflamed by the measles virus.'

'But they'll be able to treat her in hospital? Give her something to kill the virus?'

I didn't want to tell her, yet again, that there was no way of treating the virus.

'They'll be able to give her fluids – she's so dehydrated,' I explained. 'And they will be able to do more tests, to see if she has a bacterial infection as well as measles. If she has, then they'll be able to give her antibiotics.'

I rang the paediatrician on call at the local hospital and explained the situation.

I knew having a child with such an infectious disease could cause all sorts of problems for the hospital.

'I don't think we've got a spare bed in a side room,' he started. 'Are you sure you can't keep her at home?'

I resisted the urge to get a bit shirty with him. 'No, she's dehydrated, she needs fluids and, even though I know you can't treat viral meningitis, I need a paediatrician to look at her. Please.'

'OK, well, send her up to A&E. But warn the mother there may be a bed problem, that she may have a long wait, and that they may have to go to a different hospital. I won't ask why the poor kid hasn't had her MMR – I blame the *Daily Mail.* By the way, don't you write for them?'

I could hear from his tone of voice that he felt I was to blame for the whole miserable scenario but I didn't want to get into a row with him. I just wanted Fleur to get some expert care.

'Dr Rosemary, how serious is this? Should I call Tristran, her father, and get him out of work?' Julia enquired. The question surprised me. I had assumed she would definitely want to call her husband. 'Only I've been playing down how serious this is. You see, he wanted her to have the MMR. We've had huge rows about it. He said it was just a load of media hype and I was being stupid . . .' I could see tears welling up in her eyes.

I put my arm around her shoulder.

'Julia, there are loads of mothers like you who have been scared, who have looked at their perfectly healthy baby and been worried about doing harm. Don't beat yourself up about it – you did what you thought was best. Now just get some overnight things together, while I organise an ambulance. I don't think Fleur can travel in a car. And to answer your question, I don't think the situation is immediately life threatening, but yes, you should call her father.'

The Power of the Press

I was full of worry as I drove back to my surgery. I fervently hoped Fleur made a full recovery – not just for her sake, but for the sake of her parents' marriage.

I got a fax from the hospital to say she had been admitted to the A and E department but, as usual, I didn't get any further updates from the hospital. Trying to find out what has happened to patients who have been admitted to hospital can take ages. It meant locating which ward they were in, then ringing the ward and finding someone senior enough to be able to give details. The reality was that neither I, nor the receptionists, had time.

So I was apprehensive when I saw that one of my phone consultations listed at the end of morning surgery was to Julia.

I went down to reception before I rang. I wanted to know if anyone had heard anything. Was Fleur OK? Was she home, or had something dreadful happened?'

Like me, everyone was in the dark.

I picked up the phone with considerable trepidation.

'Hello, Dr Leonard, thank you for phoning. Have you heard from the hospital?'

'No.' Help, I thought, what's happened?

'I thought that might be the case. Fleur's coming home tomorrow.' I breathed a huge sigh of relief. 'It was measles meningitis, just like you said. She's actually recovered very well, but there seems to be a problem with her hearing. The doctors aren't sure how long this will carry on. I thought you might be able to tell me?'

I had to think fast. I knew ear problems and hearing loss could be a complication of measles, but that was all. I didn't know if it was likely to be temporary or permanent.

'Julia, I'm not an expert on this and don't know much about it. Let me have a chat to her consultant, then I'll get back to you.'

The consultant was helpful – and the moment I'd spoken to him I understood his reticence.

'Like most measles cases Fleur's ears were very inflamed and because she had meningitis, we put her on antibiotics, just as a precaution really. But her hearing went suddenly and the tests we've done so far suggest it's nerve damage. We really need to wait a bit longer to know whether it's permanent.'

This wasn't something I could discuss with Julia over the phone. I rang her and said I needed to go through some diagrams of the ear to explain what was going on. I suggested that, if possible, she should leave Fleur with a friend. I thought it better I see her alone.

I could see she had lost weight when she came in. She was always trim, now she looked gaunt and thin.

'Sit yourself down. You've had an awful time.'

'Never mind me, it's Fleur I'm worried about. Did you manage to speak to anyone at the hospital?'

'Yes.' I dug out an anatomy text book with a cross section diagram of the ear. I explained that there were two possibilities – if the middle section of the ear had been infected and filled with fluid, as it often is, it would prevent movement of the three tiny bones that transmit sound waves from the ear drum. The fluid would eventually drain away and hearing would improve. But, if the loss of hearing was due to damage to the nerve that took the sound messages to the brain, then it could well be permanent.

'The tests done on Fleur in hospital suggest it's a mixture of the two.' I tried to be positive. 'While she was in hospital her ear drums were very red, which means there was some inflammation in the middle ear. We just need to wait a few weeks to see how much her hearing improves. But there is a possibility she will always have some hearing loss. If that's the case, we'll get her fixed up with one of the new tiny digital hearing aids.'

'Oh my God. Poor Fleur. And Tristran will be even more furious with me. He can barely bring himself to speak to me as it is. He blames me and thinks I'm a silly fool. Which of course I am. This is all my fault.'

I felt very sorry for her. 'Would it help if I had a word with him?' I offered. 'What Fleur needs now is love and support from her parents.'

'Would you? He might just be a little more under-standing if the news came from you.'

I'd never met Tristran – in fact, though he was registered with us, he'd only ever been to the surgery once in the six years since the family had moved into the area. I was aware when I picked up the phone, later on that day, that the call might be a bit tricky. One of my typical understatements.

'Tristran, it's Dr Leonard, from the surgery.'

'Ah you're the one who agreed with my wife that the MMR was dangerous, aren't you?'

'Errr, no. I had several conversations with Julia about the MMR and tried to persuade her to let Fleur have the vaccine.'

'But you didn't, did you? You couldn't have explained properly how safe these vaccines are, could you? Why didn't you just go ahead and give her the jab?'

'We can't go giving vaccines without parental consent—'

'So why didn't you call me? I'd have given permission.'

Well, why didn't you come down to the surgery with your wife, then, I thought to myself. But saying it out loud wasn't going to help.

'Julia did say she was going to discuss it with you—'

'But Fleur didn't have the vaccine. And that's not just Julia's fault. It's your fault, too – you should have done a better job at persuading her to let Fleur be vaccinated.'

'Tristran, can we discuss her hearing? Some of her deafness may be due to residual fluid in her middle ear, which will drain away. But there is a possibility that the nerve has been damaged.'

'And that means she'll have to wear hearing aids?'

'Yes, I'm afraid so.'

'I'm never going to be able to forgive Julia for this – it's all her fault.'

'I know you are angry with her—'

'And you.'

'Yes, I understand that, but being angry now isn't going to help Fleur . . .'

'I suppose you're going to suggest I go and "talk" to someone. Have some counselling or therapy? Well, I'll tell you now, Dr Leonard, I don't need any advice – especially from you. If you'd done your job properly none of this would have happened.'

And with that the line went dead.

So much for trying to help.

Julia came in with Fleur a month later. Fleur was her usual happy self but Julia, if anything, looked thinner than before and was downcast.

'Could you check her ears, please? I don't think her hearing has improved very much, and we're going back to the hospital tomorrow, and I just want to be sure that it isn't wax, or that they aren't still infected.'

'Of course.' I asked Fleur to come over to the side of my desk, but she clearly didn't hear me. At all. I hoped my shock didn't show. And there was nothing in her ear canals. No inflammation. No wax.

'How much does she hear at home?' I asked Julia.

'Very, very little. I'm just hoping that hearing aids will help.'

'And how are things with Tristran?' Normally, I wouldn't have this type of conversation with a young child present, but Fleur was immersed in the box of toys behind my desk and I now knew she couldn't hear what we were saying.

'It's dreadful. He just won't let me forget that this is all my fault. I think he hates me – every night he just keeps reminding me what a bloody fool I've been. I just don't know what to say to him – nothing I say can put it right. I hope he'll come to the hospital tomorrow – maybe the doctor there will be able to calm him down a bit. But, of course, he's right to be angry – it is all my stupid fault.'

She was a broken woman.

'Julia, you need to stay strong for Fleur – to help her through this, no matter how little she can hear.'

'If only I had listened to you about the vaccine. Are people still refusing to have it?'

'Not as many as before, but yes. And we've had another couple of cases of measles round here.'

'Well, I can't put right the wrong I've done, but if ever you need someone to say how dangerous measles can be, let me know.'

The letter I received from the hospital confirmed that Fleur had severe sensorineural hearing loss – deafness due to damage to the nerves that take the sound messages to the ear. The digital aid she was being fitted with wouldn't return her hearing back to where it was, but hopefully it would mean that she could live a fairly normal life.

A couple of months later, I had a call from one of the journalists at *BBC Breakfast*. 'Hi, Rosemary, I wonder if you can help. The latest measles statistics have just been published and they've shown a big rise in the number of cases. Can you come on and talk about it on tomorrow's programme?'

'Sure. Tell me, do the statistics show there a lot here where I'm working, in south-east London? We've had several cases in our surgery.'

'Yes, it's a real hot spot. And, on that note, I don't suppose you know anyone who could come on and talk about it first hand? A parent maybe?'

Normally I'm reluctant to involve any of my patients in my media work – I like to keep the two completely separate. But, bearing in mind what Julia had said, I thought it was worthwhile giving her a call.

'Julia, you know what you said about speaking out about measles – how about talking about it on *BBC Breakfast*? Please don't feel you need to do it for me – only do it if you want to for yourself. I don't mind one way or the other.' Which was true – the BBC could always find someone else. I didn't want her to feel obliged or pressurized into anything.

'Yes, I'd like to do it, Rosemary. To stop people getting sucked into the hysteria about the vaccine like I was. But I'll have to ask Tristran. Things still aren't good. I don't want to aggravate him in any way.'

'No problem. But as usual with the BBC they'll need to know quite soon, as they would like someone for tomorrow. How long will you need?'

'An hour or so?'

'Fine. I'll give you my mobile number so you can call me direct.'

She rang me back, very conveniently, at the end of morning surgery.

'Sorry, Rosemary, can't do it. Tristran won't have it. Says how can I possibly think of showing myself up to be such an ignorant fool on national TV. And, of course, he's right.'

'No problem.' It genuinely wasn't. But I was concerned. 'Julia, how are things between the two of you?'

'Don't go there.'

'No better?'

'Worse. To be honest, I'm not sure how much more I can take. He reminds me every day that it's my fault that Fleur is deaf. I know neither of us will ever get over this, but I've somehow got to pull myself together and be positive, for her sake. And I can't while he's being, well, so vile to me.'

'Any chance that he would go to some sort of counselling with you?'

'No chance at all. He says that everything is my fault – it's nothing to do with him.'

'Julia, how were things between the two of you before all this business?' I wondered if he had always been this intransigent.

'Not great, but OK. He's never been an easy man. Always very sure of himself. But I think he loved me, and he could be kind to me. That's all gone now.'

I wished I could somehow get the message across to Tristan that it takes two to make a relationship work, but after my last encounter with him, I didn't think it was advisable.

I brought it up at the next practice meeting. It turned out he'd rung David about Fleur's hearing aids, and it wasn't just me he was angry with. It seemed he felt the whole practice had been at fault for not ensuring she had her MMR.

'I just don't see what we can do,' I said . 'I can see the marriage falling apart. Which is sad for all of them.'

A week later, Julia came into the surgery while Fleur was at school.

'Tristran had another outburst over the weekend,' she explained, 'shouting and screaming at me. I've had enough. I'm going to take Fleur at stay with my mother for a few weeks down in Sussex. I've checked with the school and I'll teach her myself till things are more settled. Maybe if we go away for a few weeks, Tristran will calm down a bit.'

It seemed a very sensible plan and I fully expected that I'd see her again soon.

But I didn't. That was the end of the marriage. She never came back. She stayed down in Sussex and started to make a new life for herself and her daughter. And, as always happens, once a patient has moved to another GP's list, I lost contact.

I only hope they are thriving , and are happy.

* * *

Andrew Wakefield was found guilty of serious professional misconduct by the General Medical Council and was struck off the medical register in 2010. He is no longer allowed to practice as a doctor in the United Kingdom. *The Lancet* fully retracted his original paper shortly afterwards. There were thirteen co-authors of the original report and ten of them have disowned it.

I wonder if any of them have any idea how many lives they have wrecked.

CHAPTER THIRTEEN

THE DRIVER

It was going to be another rushed morning.

I'd done one appearance on *BBC Breakfast* at 6.40am and was approaching my beloved little hatchback parked outside BBC Television Centre in west London when my mobile rang. It was the editor of *Breakfast*.

'Rosemary, there have been a lot of emails coming in about your story, can you stay on and answer some of them at ten past eight?'

I had a surgery starting at 9am at my practice in south London, and I knew I'd be cutting it fine to get back in time for the first patient, but I thought it was possible. 'Sure, no problem. I'll come back to the studio.'

How wrong I was.

I knew I wasn't going to make it as soon as I pulled on to the A40, to be faced with a mile of stationary traffic. At 8.50am I was still stuck on the north side of the river. I rang the surgery (a hands-free kit is one of the most useful investments a GP can make!) to apologise – to both the patients who would be kept waiting and to the receptionists who would be on the front line taking the flak.

'Oh, don't worry, Rosemary, we'll cope. If they can't wait, though, can we move some of them to later on today?'

I tried to practise what I preach as I waited at yet another set of red traffic lights. 'Don't get uptight,' I kept saying to myself. 'It's not going to help. Just keep calm, no one is going to die – hopefully.' I knew that if someone was really ill in my absence the surgery staff and other doctors could deal with it. Nevertheless, I could feel my pulse rate increasing and when I finally arrived twenty minutes late, there was sweat dripping from my brow. One of the side effects of TV appearances is the vast quantity of make-up that they put on you and, unfortunately, the sweat on my face was taking a good deal of that make-up with it – the mascara smudging under my eyes. Not a good look.

'Large cup of coffee?' asked Lizzy as I dashed passed reception.

'Oh, please, you saviour.'

I called in my first patient. I knew Betty well. A sprightly seventy-eight-year-old, she'd been having trouble with arthritis in her knees for the last five years. She'd resisted having any surgical treatment because she'd been caring for her husband, who had died of lung cancer the previous year. She was dressed immaculately, as usual, in a tweed skirt and purple cashmere jumper, with a double strand of pearls (obviously real ones) around her neck, matching her large pearl earrings.

'I know you're running late, so I'll be quick. I think the time has come to do something about my right knee. It gave way again during my ballroom dancing session last week and I've had a couple of falls since then. I don't have to look after George any more, but my older sister lives miles away and getting to her isn't easy when I'm not fit. I reckon if I get it sorted now I'll be right as rain in a few weeks.'

I was glad she was finally agreeing to see a specialist – an X-ray I'd done before George had died had shown severe arthritis in her knee, so much so I was amazed that she seemed to be able to ignore the pain. But her timings were wildly ambitious, so I outlined a rough timetable for her. First of all she would have to wait for an outpatient appointment, and then there would be several months' wait before she had her operation. And if, as I suspected, she needed the joint replaced, she would be laid up for more than just a few weeks.

'What if I went private?' she asked.

'Have you got insurance?'

'No – I used to, but as I got older the premiums got more and more expensive. So I cancelled the policy and have been putting the money in a high-interest account instead – to pay for things like this.'

An increasing number of my financially better-off patients were taking this line. I didn't blame them – as you get older the health insurance premiums tend to rise significantly year-on-year.

'Even so – it will cost you a small fortune. Why don't I refer you to see the consultant on the NHS and he'll advise you on what exactly you need done and how much it will cost. Then you can decide what you want to do.' Even if she had the money, I didn't like the idea of her using her savings for something that could be done perfectly well on the NHS.

'No, I'd prefer to see the specialist as soon as possible. After all, I can't take my savings with me, and George and I provided perfectly well for our children. I want to be fit to look after my sister as soon as possible.'

I wrote a referral letter for her to see Mike Wilkinson, the consultant who specialised in knees at the local hospital, and gave her his telephone number to make an appointment.

'He is good, isn't he? He will be able to see me quickly, won't he?' she seemed determined to get her knee sorted out as soon as possible.

'If I had a problem with my knees, he's the person I would see. He's sorted out lots of my patients and they have all been very happy with his care. I also like him because he's not "knife happy" – he won't operate unless he really thinks you need surgery, and that's not always the case in the private sector. I trust him completely. I know he's a keen dinghy sailor but his boat isn't on the water yet and his children aren't on school holidays yet, so I imagine he'll be able to see you in the next week or so.'

'And if he can't?'

Goodness, she was clearly determined not to hang around with getting her operation done, I thought to myself.

'Then I'll find someone else.'

I didn't hear anything more for ten days, when a letter arrived from Mike. He confirmed that Betty's knee was so worn that the best option was for it to be replaced, and this was planned for the following week. So it was with considerable surprise that she turned up in my surgery just three days before her operation.

She wasn't happy.

'I've just had a letter from the police. Another three points for speeding. Ridiculous. They say I was doing fifty in a thirty limit.' Goodness me, that is pretty quick, I thought to myself. 'Well, I don't think I was. But if I was going a bit fast, it must have been because of my knee. I'm going to appeal. Can you write a letter confirming I have a knee problem?'

I could see this wasn't going to be easy. There were two things I was about to say that were unlikely to make her any happier. Firstly, no, I couldn't write such a letter – having a dodgy knee is no excuse for breaking the speed limit. Secondly, if your knee is sufficiently dodgy that you can't control the pedals, you probably shouldn't be driving at all.

'Betty, you say you've got *another* three points. How many have you got already?'

'Oh, I've only got three so far. But it's just so ridiculous. I was driving perfectly safely.'

'Betty, having a dodgy knee isn't an excuse for going too fast. If anything, it means you shouldn't be driving at all, especially as that's the leg that controls the accelerator. If you really think that's the reason you were going too fast, then you ought not to drive until you've had the operation and are fully recovered.'

My advice went down like a lead balloon. This was, as expected, not what she wanted or expected to hear.

'So there's nothing I can do about the points?'

'I don't think so. And please, take care. Perhaps you should think about stopping driving until after the operation.'

'Oh, don't be silly, Dr Leonard, I can drive perfectly well. Never had an accident. I was just going at a perfectly sensible speed but got caught by one of those stupid cameras.'

A discharge letter arrived three weeks later confirming her operation had been straightforward and that she was now back at home. She phoned me a couple of days later.

'A couple of things, Dr Leonard. I need some more painkillers – could you arrange that for me?'

'Of course. How is your knee? Is it very painful? You were sent home with two different lots of painkillers – which ones do you want?'

'Oh, not the strong ones. I just need something to take the edge off the pain while I do my exercises. I was hoping to come down to the surgery but I can't walk quite that far yet. Which brings me to the second thing – when can I drive? I need to get down to see my sister.'

Ah yes. The driving. A little voice in my head said, 'Tread with care, Rosemary.'

'Betty, while I'm all for you making a quick recovery, you have got to take things gently. You can't drive until you are confident you are completely in control of the car. That means being able to do an emergency stop without any pain. The minimum time it takes is a month, but for most people it takes at least six weeks.'

'Six weeks?!' she shrieked down the phone.

'Yes,' I tried to answer in my most calm, reassuring manner.

'Well, we'll see about that.' And with that, the line went dead.

Just under a month later I spotted her behind the wheel of her Nissan Micra, staring intently ahead. So much for the six-week warning – well, that was her prerogative. I just fervently hoped she could do an emergency stop, especially as she was clearly going more than the thirty-mile-an-hour limit and was passing perilously close to the cars parked on the left-hand side. I was concerned but there wasn't anything that I could really do about it. I'm a doctor, not a traffic officer. I didn't have enough evidence to say she was unfit to drive and I was well aware that there were plenty of others on the roads who drove just as fast – if not more so – than her. If anything, her new knee should have improved her driving. My knowledge of her points made me suspect that she took a lax attitude to speed limits anyway, regardless of the state of her knees.

I didn't see Betty again for several months. When she next appeared, it was to discuss her other knee – the left.

'It's giving way and last week it locked. I couldn't move it. It caused a bit of a problem – couldn't change gear. I had to drive all the way back from my sister's in second.'

Alarm bells started going off in my head. This lady had knees that clearly impaired her ability to drive. But getting her to stop driving was like telling a squirrel to stop hiding nuts.

'It sounds like the cartilage is worn in that one as well. We need to get you to see Mr Wilkinson again. NHS this time?'

'No, I'll go privately. The sooner I get it done, the better. I can't keep driving fifty miles in one gear. I don't suppose it's terribly good for the engine.'

'Betty, promise me, please, if the knee locks again that you stop driving until you've had it seen to. It really isn't safe to drive if you can't use the clutch.'

A couple of weeks later, a letter arrived from Mike confirming Betty's left knee had been replaced as well. Having both knees replaced is quite a common scenario – it's rare to get arthritis in just one knee. But most patients wait a bit longer between their operations. This was one lady in a hurry. She came into the surgery a few weeks later.

'This left leg is still bit painful. Can't move it quite as well as the other one. Can you just give it the once-over?'

I examined her knee. The scars had healed but the movement was certainly very restricted.

'You just need to give it a bit more time. Make sure you do the exercises on the sheet you were given when you left hospital, and I'm sure some more movement will return in due course. I'll arrange some more physiotherapy for you as well.'

I had assumed that Betty was making her way around walking slowly, using public transport and getting lifts from friends. Her left knee had perhaps thirty degrees of movement – there was no way she was safe behind the wheel of her manual Micra.

It hadn't occurred to me that she might have driven to the surgery. It was Lizzy who told me as we were waiting for the kettle to boil in the kitchen.

'You know Betty, with the two new knees? Should she be driving?'

'Oh god. Please tell me she's not.'

'Only from my desk upstairs I've a bird's eye view of the road and she seemed to be having problems parking. She stalled at least twice and I'm sure she bumped the car in front. Her parking was pretty atrocious – she just left the car half out in the road, with the front wing sticking out. It's a miracle no one hit it.'

It was clear another phone call was in order.

'Betty, as I said before, please don't drive until you have full control of the car.'

'Oh, it's all right, Dr Leonard, I've decided to get an automatic. That way I won't have to use my left knee. The other one's as right as rain now.'

'Promise me, please, you won't drive until you have your new car?'

She skirted the question, 'I'm not as dangerous as you think I am, you know, but I do realise my left knee is a problem.'

'So you won't drive?'

'OK, then, if you say so – but only until I have my new car.'

At present, drivers can keep their licence until they reach the age of seventy. Then they have to reapply for a licence every three years. There is a lengthy list of questions about medical conditions that might disqualify you from driving on the application form but, ultimately, it's up the person to decide to tick – or not – any of the boxes. You don't have to undergo any type of medical test, and no one checks whether you are lying or not. There is no age limit on driving, so if someone considers themselves fit to do so, then they can drive on their hundredth birthday.

To be fair, the system generally works well. Statistics show that eight per cent of Britain's drivers are over seventy, yet they are only involved in four per cent of crashes resulting in injury. Meanwhile, fifteen per cent of drivers are in their teens or twenties, and for them that same figure is thirty-four per cent. And driving does give many older people vital independence. My own mother, living in a tiny village in deepest Dorset, where there is only one bus a week, would be stranded without a car. She would hate to be reliant on other people to get out and about for her shopping and her social life.

I didn't see Betty again until a winter's morning some eighteen months later. She came in with her right arm in a sling.

'Oh, I slipped on the ice, and I've gone and broken my wrist. Colles fracture is what they called it. Real nuisance. Can't do much cooking, can't do the ironing, but the real problem is I can't drive. I can't hold the steering wheel. I've asked the doctors at the hospital when they think I will be able to get behind the wheel again, but they won't give me a straight answer. Says it depends how long it takes to get my grip back properly.'

'They're right, Betty, there is no "straight answer" on this one. It's all a question of safety. You've got to be patient.'

'Well, I can't hang around. I have to go and see my sister at least once a week and I keep having to ask my neighbours to get my shopping in. I need to do it myself. I've never been good at lists. I like to see what's on the shelves and what's on special offer.'

I sympathised and silently agreed with her. As my sons will testify, I've never been any good at planning meals either.

It was Lizzy, once again, who informed me that Betty was behind the wheel within a few weeks. I had visions of Betty, right arm still in sling, doing battle with an automatic Nissan Micra on the streets of south London. A truly terrifying prospect.

'She was at the butcher's yesterday and she got in the car and pulled off. She never seemed to check if anyone was coming – she didn't look in her mirrors or anything. A poor cyclist was almost sent flying; it could have been really nasty.'

No one wanted to stop Betty driving and take away her independence, but we didn't want her involved in a nasty crash either. It was agreed I would talk to her about her driving.

She came in again for a check-up a couple of weeks later and, treading on eggshells, I broached the subject as tactfully as I could.

'Betty, what with two new knees and a recently broken arm, driving can't be as easy for you as it used to be.'

'Dr Leonard, you are for ever going on at me about my driving. It's bad enough having the police on my back, giving me fines and points.'

'More points, Betty?'

'I must remember about the camera on the A2, on the way to Sittingbourne. Got caught out by that again recently. I'm up to nine now.' She said with a tone of resentment. 'Still, got a few more spare. I do hate the way this country is so Big Brotherish now. Everyone's spying on me – all the time. Including, it would seem,' she said with a glare, 'you.'

'Betty, I just have your best interests at heart. I don't want you having an accident and injuring yourself, or someone else. How about taking a refresher course?' I added, trying to offer some friendly advice.

'Refresher course? What on earth do you mean? I didn't need any lessons to learn to drive – and I don't now.'

I knew it was common for people in the forties and fifties to be taught to drive by their family, but I thought most had a lesson or two just before their test.

'But what about passing your test? Surely you had some formal instruction before that?'

'I've never taken a driving test in my life,' she retorted, as if passing a driving test was something to be disdainful of.

It was only then that I remembered my late father hadn't taken a formal test either, and she was born in the same year as him. He'd learnt to drive in the war, when driving tests were suspended. He'd been given a provisional licence, which he'd been able to convert automatically to a full one, with no questions asked, in 1957. Betty had done exactly the same. But, unlike my father, who had gone on to pass his advanced test and become a member of the Institute of Advanced Motorists, Betty had continued to drive how she always had done. Badly. It was small miracle that she'd never had a major accident.

I wasn't sure what, if anything I could do. Later that day, when surgery had finished and I had a quiet half hour, I pulled out the document that gives doctors guidelines on medical standards on Fitness to Drive. I checked through the sections – neurological, kidney and circulatory disorders, diabetes, psychiatric disorders, eye problems, even drug and alcohol misuse. Betty didn't fit into any of those, and I didn't think she qualified as 'disabled' either. And, though she was undoubtedly stubborn, I had no evidence that she was losing her memory or was, as the booklet called it 'cognitively impaired'. I couldn't see that I had any real medical grounds to tell her to stop driving.

It was a few months later, during afternoon surgery when I heard the sound of screeching brakes and then the horrid crunch of metal. There had obviously been an accident on the road outside. Along with Lizzy, who was on reception, I dashed out of the front door of the surgery, fervently hoping that no one had been hurt. I was aware that it was 4.30pm, and a lot of children – including mine – were coming home from school on foot and on bicycles.

We could see there was a commotion just along the road and, as we approached, it became clear that two cars had been involved. It seemed fairly obvious what had happened: A blue Nissan Micra had gone into the back of a large silver BMW estate. The Micra had come off significantly worse and, while the BMW looked a few years old, the Micra looked almost brand new. A quick check of the respective number plates confirmed this.

However, as we got closer to the accident I saw that one of the drivers was Betty. I immediately knew which of the drivers she was – Betty had clearly replaced her old red Micra with a new automatic blue one. The other driver was a middle-aged lady and there were two children strapped in the back of the BMW.

The lady was shouting at Betty, telling her that she was driving far too close, hadn't left any stopping distance and it was all her fault. Betty remained indignant and her defence seemed to be, 'What was that other car doing stopping so suddenly.' I could understand the other driver's anger – Betty appeared to have ploughed with some force into the back of the lady's car. She was taking her children home from school. If it had been me, I'd have been angry, too.

I quickly checked to see if everyone was OK, checking the children first, then the other driver, then Betty. Once I'd got to Betty she said she was fine, but I could see that she didn't want to bear weight on her right leg. It transpired her leg had smashed into the underside of the dashboard in the impact and it was clearly hurting her. She didn't want to make a fuss, but I insisted she come into the surgery for a check-up.

The BMW could be driven away, with just the back bumper and tailgate noticeably damaged. Betty's Micra was crumpled all the way along the bonnet and front wings, and both front wheels were pushed out to one side. The car had crumpled under the impact as it was designed to do. As she came into the surgery, I didn't need to mention driving to Betty, her car was probably a write-off so it was unlikely she'd be getting behind the wheel any time soon. Thank goodness there had been no serious injury, but perhaps this accident was a blessing in disguise, I thought. Perhaps now Betty would stop driving.

But two months later was another incident. Again Lizzy saw it as she was sitting by the top office window.

'Betty's just driven her car on to the pavement. She doesn't seem to have proper control over where she's going. She nearly hit a group of children waiting outside the newsagent.'

I brought it up again at the next practice meeting.

'I haven't got a definite medical reason for stopping her driving,' I explained, 'but there seems to be no doubt she's dangerous. She's an accident waiting to happen, and perhaps the next one won't be quite as minor. Anyone could get hurt.' Including, I thought silently, my own sons, or their friends.

I asked Betty to come into the surgery, on the pretext of doing a routine check on her knees, which we now did, rather than the hospital. I told her I thought she should stop driving until she had done a proper course to prove that she was fit to do so, or I would report her to the DVLA. I told her my reasons – her safety and that of others.

She was furious, telling me I was an interfering madam. She admitted her right knee had been hurting and was stiff, and that was why she had driven on to the pavement. But she was going to have some physiotherapy and it would soon be back to normal again. Certainly, she wasn't going to stop driving. She'd never hurt anyone (except herself, I thought) and wasn't going to do so now. She said that I didn't know what I was talking about. And she was fed up with my domineering attitude.

'No good having a doctor who is trying to clip my wings the whole time,' she proclaimed. 'You're not going to have me sitting in a chair doing nothing.'

She told me she was leaving the surgery and going to register with another local practice where she knew the doctors would be more helpful and sympathetic.

Knowing her address, I knew which practice she would be going to. I knew them well – it was where I was registered myself – and I rang up the manager to warn them why she had left us. 'She's OK, really, just a dreadful driver.' And then, very sadly, I wrote to the DVLA. Once the decision had been made, I didn't want to wait any longer. I knew I was taking away her independence but I felt I had no option. I'd given her enough chances and the reasoning I had given to her was to stop her hurting anyone – and that could happen at any time.

The very next day Lizzy phoned through from reception.

'It's Alan on the phone, the manager from the neighbouring practice. Wants to speak to you.'

'Hello, Alan, how can I help you?'

'Rosemary, I thought I ought to tell you straight away. That patient of yours, Betty, she came here to register this morning.'

'Oh?'

'She arrived with a bit of bang. Drove straight into the front of the senior partner's car. Made a right old mess of it. Reckon it could be a write off. He's not very happy . . .'

'I bet he's not. And Betty? Anyone hurt?'

'No, no one hurt. Betty's OK – just. But her car's not. It's in an even worse state than the doctor's!'

'I don't think her insurance company are going to be too happy either. That's the second major prang she's had in a month.'

'She didn't say anything about you being right, but she seemed quite shaken up. And she did mumble something about doing an older driver's refresher course before she got behind the wheel again.'

I never heard from Betty again. I was actually quite fond of her and would have welcomed her back as a patient, if she had decided she didn't want to stay with the new surgery. But I suspected, correctly, that she was too proud to come back and say I had been right all along. I later discovered, at a local GPs' meeting, that she had apparently stopped driving. She stayed with the new surgery, avoiding the doctor whose car she had pranged, if possible, but had to be taken there by a friend. That saddened me – deciding not to drive meant she had lost some of the independence that was so important to her. But maybe she knew it was too late to teach an old dog new tricks.

CHAPTER FOURTEEN

FIT FOR NOTHING

It was a balmy Monday morning in June, a warm breeze was gently lifting the curtains in my bedroom and the room was already lit with hefty stripes of sunshine. It was only 6am so the day was destined to become a scorcher.

However, all this was a bit wasted on me in my present physical state.

I peeled back the duvet and wondered how best to move without wincing. Sitting up was the necessary first stage and my abdomen contracted in protest. I swung round and tentatively wriggled my bare toes on the carpet. So far, so good.

Then, far too over-confidently and far too fast, I stood up and pain shot through my body. It hurt to bend my legs and my bottom felt as if it had been scraped with wire wool. I made my way to the bathroom, adopting a rather ludicrously stiff walk to minimise bending my knees, and turned on the shower. Bliss. The needles of steaming water did not ease all the aches and pains, but my body did experience a little bit of the rebirth it needed to cope with the long working day ahead.

I felt as if I'd been in a road accident but I had merely been on a bike ride. A pretty long one, admittedly; it was something I do only once a year with totally inadequate training beforehand. No wonder my body was objecting.

I never learn. The day before, I had embarked upon the London to Brighton bike ride for the sixth time and, I reflected, it just did not get any easier.

It had started as a challenge for me and my oldest son, Thomas, who wanted to do it as soon as he was old enough. You are first allowed on the ride at the age of fourteen but until you hit sixteen you have to be accompanied by an adult and that meant me.

Held annually in June, it is Europe's biggest fund-raising cycle ride and perhaps its most popular, with 27,000 riders taking part.

The fifty-four-mile ride starts in Clapham Common in south London but exact details are not disclosed until the day, when you are given a Route Card, which also lists official refreshment stops and an emergency number should you need medical attention. Since 2006 those who complete the race also receive a well done medal.

The very first London to Brighton bike ride was held in 1976. A mere sixty riders took part and the route was a gruelling ninety-five miles. Only thirty-seven people completed it, which may be why the organisers have made it a bit more 'people friendly'.

I had started a team called Strictly Come Cycling and persuaded many of my colleagues on *BBC Breakfast* to take part with me.

The most enthusiastic recruits for this annual torture were always from the BBC weather team. Lovely Carol Kirkwood has always been very supportive and so, too, has Chris Hollins, that man of many talents, who won the nation's hearts when he won *Strictly Come Dancing* in 2009.

I am always as stiff as a board the following morning and, despite my padded cycling shorts, have to sit very gingerly on chairs and endure endless ragging from the medical practice staff as I try to walk without showing any signs of discomfort.

I persisted with the ride, partly as a physical challenge, but also because my father Gordon died of heart disease and I want to raise awareness of the British Heart Foundation, who organise the event.

Lizzy, who had worked for the surgery for years, laughed as I walked in. 'No prizes for guessing what you were doing yesterday. Extra cushion needed for your chair?'

I perched by my desk uncomfortably, trying to keep as much pressure off my bottom as possible, when Sandra came into my consulting room.

I first met Sandra when she moved to the area as a new graduate to teach classics at one of the local secondary schools. She was twenty-five, had shoulder-length, dark blonde hair and blue eyes, but I did not know her well. She had rarely come to the surgery during the two years she had been my patient. Looking through her notes I saw that her only visits had been for a cut hand that had become infected, a smear test and family planning advice. All very sensible reasons.

Her stricken face immediately alerted me that this time something was seriously wrong. She seemed to be carrying the weight of the world on her shoulders as she sat down heavily and began twiddling her hair with her right index finger. 'It's not exactly me,' she began, 'it's my father. He's had a heart attack. He's OK – they've put a stent in the blocked artery – but we're all so shocked. Dad's the last person I'd expect to have a dodgy ticker. He's never smoked, eats healthily, keeps his weight down and takes regular exercise. He puts me to shame. Thank goodness he's recovering well but it seems that his heart problem could run in the family.'

It transpired that Sandra's father had a very raised cholesterol level and that when his brother was tested, his was even higher.

'I've been told to have my cholesterol tested, too, because dad's specialist says it is almost certainly a genetic problem that could affect me.'

The blood test I arranged confirmed that Sandra's levels were way too high. Her total cholesterol was 8 mmol/l, three above the recommended upper level of 5. Her level of LDL (low-density lipoprotein), the harmful part of cholesterol that can lead to fatty deposits building up in the linings of arteries, was 5.6, when it should have been a maximum 3.

Blood cholesterol comes from two sources – a quarter of it from food. When anyone comes in with a reading that is too high, the first thing to consider is their diet. Sometimes just cutting out foods high in saturated fat, such as butter, cream, pastries and fatty meats, is all that is required to bring levels back down to normal. However, I thought it highly unlikely that levels as high as these in a slim twenty-five-year-old were due to a bad diet, and when we talked through what Sandra ate, it was clear there was very little room for improvement.

'I probably eat more than five daily portions of fruit and vegetables,' she said. 'I love being creative with salads and always start my day with a home-made fruit smoothie.'

She had been brought up never to add salt to her food and, as a consequence, could not stand the taste of ready meals which use salt as a cheap source of bulk and flavouring, nor did she like crisps which are extremely high in salt content. 'I'm very disciplined,' she said. 'No matter how tired I am after work, I always cook fresh food for myself, preferably organic, even though I live alone. My one weakness is chocolate but I try to keep it as a treat.'

The remaining three-quarters of cholesterol in the blood are made in the liver, and this is where genetics can come into play. A faulty gene means that in some families the liver is programmed to produce large amounts of LDL. One in 500 people carry this gene and, unfortunately, even if their diet is very low in fat, their cholesterol level will still be high. The only way to bring it back to normal is with medication.

I advised Sandra that she needed to take a statin. This group of drugs work by reducing the amount of cholesterol produced by the liver. Sandra wanted advice on what else she could do to reduce her future risk of heart problems.

She had never smoked and we calculated her BMI (Body Mass Index) to be an ideal 22 so there was no room for improvement there.

Excess alcohol can also increase the risk of heart disease but Sandra said that she drank alcohol only when she went out with friends and reckoned it came to around ten units a week. 'I'm a bit of a cheap date,' she said. 'I feel high as a kite after a couple of drinks and I don't like the feeling of losing control you get with too much alcohol. I had a horrible experience with booze at university once and I don't want to go there again.'

Government guidelines recommend that women drink no more than two to three units of alcohol a day, the equivalent of a 175ml glass of wine, and a new initiative, prompted by concerns about binge drinking and addiction, is now urging people to have two alcohol-free days a week.

Sometimes doctors mentally double whatever a patient says they drink, but I had no reason to think Sandra was being dishonest and her consumption was well below the guidelines.

But I had a surprise when we came to questions about exercise. Sandra was so slim that I thought she'd be a gym bunny or take part in regular sport but she looked a tad shamefaced.

'I don't do anything,' she admitted. 'I'm a complete couch potato. I just hate exercise but I suppose I should rethink that now.'

I explained that even if her cholesterol level was well controlled by medication, which would minimise her risk of heart disease, regular exercise was an important part of staying healthy.

'You are beautifully slim now,' I said, 'but, believe me, I know all about this – you will find it much more difficult to maintain your good figure as you get older without being more physically active.'

A determined look came over Sandra's face. 'Dad's always done a charity sporting event of some sort every year and he probably won't be able to this year, so I'll do one instead.'

I agreed it was an excellent plan and told her about the ride I'd done the day before.

'I like the idea of that,' said Sandra. 'Also, as it's in aid of a heart charity it would be appropriate and Dad would be so proud of me. Cycling sounds a lot more fun than jogging. I tried doing that once with a friend and it bored me witless. I hated it. I don't know how those people do the marathon – it's the last thing I'd ever want to do – but I could be persuaded to ride a bike.'

As with all patients I start on statins, I saw her again three months later to check how she was getting on with the medication, especially checking if she was having any side effects. She reported back that she didn't feel any different, and a blood test confirmed her cholesterol level had fallen to 4.5, with an LDL of 2.7. I advised her to continue with the medication indefinitely, though warned her she would need to stop it if she became pregnant.

The next time I met Sandra was not in the surgery, but unexpectedly a year later, on the London to Brighton bike ride. I was on the winding road up Ditchling Beacon – the calf-killing ascent has to be tackled when you have already cycled fifty miles and it's not for the faint-hearted.

Ditchling Beacon is legendary among cyclists. It rises to 248 metres in just over 1.6 kilometres (one mile) and the road sweeps from side to side and around a number of sharp bends.

It is the highest point in East Sussex and the third highest on the South Downs, and although it will test your legs to their limit, the views from this Iron Age hill fort site, once you reach the summit, are spectacular.

Despite vowing each year that I would manage to cycle all the way up, yet again my fitness levels had failed me. Both Thomas and William, and some of their friends, were doing the ride, and had inevitably made rude remarks as

I'd been unable to keep up with them and dismounted. I was puffing badly as I pushed my bike up the hill when Sandra cycled effortlessly past me.

'Doctor Leonard! I wondered if I'd see you on the ride,' she cried out, obviously not suffering from lack of breath herself. 'Do excuse me but I'm not going to stop or I'll never get going again – but I'll see you at the top.'

I felt demoralised. A few months ago Sandra had never even ridden a bike and look at her now, while I had struggled for years. Oh to be young.

We met outside the row of portacabin ladies' loos. As always on this ride, I was amused by the reversed status of the queues for the conveniences – a long one for the gents and a very short one for the ladies – a reflection of the male domination of this ride.

I wondered whether I was in for an ear-bashing for giving Sandra the idea of taking part in something so gruelling, but far from it. 'Look at that amazing view,' she exclaimed, surveying the wonderful vista across the South Downs. 'I am having THE most wonderful day and loving every minute of it.'

'What, even that hill?' I asked. I loathe Ditchling Beacon.

'Oh yes, that was just a great challenge for me. I've been working hard on my fitness and I feel so much better for being more active. I've been meaning to send you a letter to say thanks for making me get off the couch. I've changed my life and it's partly due to you. Anyway, can't stop to chat for any longer as I've given myself a time target today.'

With that, Sandra leapt back on her bike and started pedalling downhill towards Brighton.

I finished the ride somewhat later than Sandra did, so we did not get a chance to talk further. As I made my way back to London in the coach, my bike stacked with loads of others in a trailer behind, I marvelled that a girl who had once never left the couch could now leave me standing on a bike.

I didn't see Sandra again until a spring morning in late March nearly two years later. I thought she looked slightly thinner than before and noticed that her complexion had lost its usual bloom. However, that wasn't so unusual at that time of year when everyone looked as if they needed a bit of sun.

'I'm sure many of your patients complain of this, and I feel a bit stupid coming to see you, Dr Leonard, but two of my friends are worried about me and have insisted I talk to you,' she said.

'What's the problem?'

'I feel crushingly tired all the time – what you doctors call TATT (tired all the time syndrome). I looked it up on the internet but it shares many symptoms with some kinds of cancer and I . . .'

'Stop right there,' I said. 'Cancer is right at the bottom of the list.' I was well aware that when patients Googled their symptoms, they always latched on to the most serious and most unlikely possible diagnosis and scared themselves senseless.

'I also read that there can be a psychological reason for this perpetual tiredness I feel but actually I'm quite happy,' Sandra continued. 'My job is going well, sleep's not a problem, I'm not stressed – so I thought I ought to check I'm not anaemic or something like that.'

Sandra had done her homework correctly. The reasons for chronic tiredness can be divided into two main groups – psychological and physical. I asked Sandra a few more questions to check her emotional state, because many patients are in denial about how stressed and anxious they actually are. Sandra, though, seemed genuinely content. 'I'm not even worried about Dad any more – he's made a great recovery and has joined a jogging group,' she said.

I made further enquiries about her sleep because individual needs vary. I reckon most people need at least seven hours a night. I've come across many patients who didn't realise they were feeling shattered because they were going to bed at midnight and getting up at 6am every working day. But Sandra was an eight-hours-a-night girl. 'I turn in after the ten o'clock news and, because I live so close to the school where I teach, I don't have to get up before seven in the morning, sometimes even later.'

I moved on to possible physical reasons. Top of the list in young women is iron deficiency, usually due to a combination of heavy periods and eating too few iron-rich foods.

If it's severe enough, iron deficiency can lead to anaemia, where there is a lack of haemoglobin, the oxygen-carrying pigment in red blood cells. That can cause profound tiredness, but even low iron stores alone can sap someone's energy.

Sandra said her monthly bleed was never very heavy but that she had now become a pescetarian – a fish-eating vegetarian – which meant she wasn't having any red meat, the richest and most easily digested source of iron. That was the likely cause, then. But I also wanted to check on the rest of her diet – sometimes just going a little short of vital nutrients – common in women who are watching their weight just a little too carefully – can cause fatigue.

'Oh, I eat really well,' she assured me. 'I pig out on salads and fresh fruit,' she said. 'I eat oily fish at least twice a week and I've become pretty ingenious with turning soya protein into tasty meals. Often my friends don't even realise they are not eating meat.'

I reflected that it wasn't often I heard of such a great diet in my area of London. I was always nagging patients to eat more healthily but Sandra seemed to be doing everything right, except that, without red meat, her iron intake might be low.

I checked for symptoms of other possible medical reasons for her tiredness. An underactive thyroid can cause fatigue but usually this is accompanied by dry skin and hair, and often weight gain, too. No, Sandra had none of those symptoms either. Tiredness can also be the first sign of diabetes, but again there were no indications of this, such as constant thirst or slightly blurred vision.

I arranged for Sandra to have the standard battery of blood tests – a full blood count, thyroid function, blood sugar levels and, most importantly for her, iron levels. I was pretty sure that this last one was likely to be the cause. But I was wrong – all the tests came back normal.

Sometimes unexplained tiredness goes away as mysteriously as it appears, and I told Sandra to leave it a couple of weeks and to come back and see me again if she still felt so exhausted.

Sure enough, she did, and said she felt even worse. 'I just feel whacked out all the time,' she told me. 'I want to nod off when I'm teaching during the day, I snooze during my lunch break and find it almost impossible to exercise in the evening. Even a short run leaves me absolutely exhausted.'

'Run?' I asked, amazed. Was this the same girl who had once said she found jogging boring and failed to understand why anyone would want to run?

'Yes,' she admitted. 'After I did the bike ride, I thought I'd try something else. So I signed up to do the three peaks – you know, the one where you climb Ben Nevis, Scarfell and Snowdon in twenty-four hours. I managed that OK, so next on my list was the London marathon. I found I got quite a buzz out of running so I've signed up to do it again this year.'

'How often do you train?'

'Oh, I used to do a few miles most days, with longer runs twice a week but I'm finding it really difficult these days.'

Sandra did look thinner and when I asked about her weight she admitted she had lost a few pounds. 'I'm making sure I eat well, though, so I think it's the running,' she said.

I checked her BMI – it was down from 22 to 20 – still in the healthy range but I warned her not to let it go any lower.

I began to wonder if something more serious was going on.

'How's your digestion? Bowels OK?' Sandra reassured me she had no problems with eating and her motions – which she passed every morning, were soft and normal coloured.

Next on the list was her gynae system.

'How about your periods? Any heavy bleeding?'

In the past, Sandra had been on the pill, but she had kept forgetting to take them. A couple of years ago I had suggested she was fitted with a Mirena coil.

'The coil has been brilliant,' she said. 'My periods have been really minimal – sometimes just a little light bleeding for a day – but for at least the past six months, I haven't had any bleeding at all. Wonderful. I know it wouldn't suit everyone, but for me and all my running it's perfect.'

Like all coils, the Mirena is fitted inside the womb but, unlike the others, it has a tiny sheath containing a synthetic version of the hormone progesterone. This is slowly released into the womb, where it thins the lining. It doesn't stop ovulation but sometimes the lining is so thin that there is simply nothing to come away when a period is due. So the fact Sandra wasn't having any periods didn't ring any alarm bells – it was actually quite normal for women with a Mirena in place.

This time I did a thorough examination, but could find nothing abnormal. In fact, Sandra seemed amazingly toned and fit. I was beginning to think her tiredness had a psychological cause after all.

I enquired about her work but she said there were no problems there; she had recently been promoted and with that had come a decent pay rise.

Next, the often dangerous territory of 'significant others'. As far as I knew, Sandra had a steady boyfriend when I fitted the coil. I asked her how the relationship was going.

'It's not,' she said. 'I dumped him last year and I've been much happier since. Honestly, Dr Leonard, I'm happy being single right now. I've still got plenty of time left to have babies. Finding Mr Right – or more realistically Mr Nearly Right – isn't an issue for me at the moment.'

Sandra genuinely did not appear to have any worries except her tiredness. And that remained a mystery.

I did some more tests, including markers for inflammation and auto-immune diseases such as lupus, which can present with tiredness. I also did a chest X-ray; London is the TB capital of Europe and, although it's more common in immigrants and drug addicts, anyone can get it – I had recently discovered a wealthy professional patient of mine had it, which had caught everyone by surprise, including me. As an afterthought, I also ticked the boxes to check Sandra's hormone levels, to be doubly sure that her Mirena coil was to blame for her lack of periods.

Once again, everything came back normal, with one exception – her hormone levels.

I had tested Sandra's levels of FSH and LH – both are produced by the pituitary gland in the brain and stimulate the ovaries to produce both oestrogen and eggs. As oestrogen levels rise, so FSH levels fall, and vice versa, which is nature's way of keeping the system in balance. The ovaries stop working at the time of the menopause and this can be detected not only by a fall in levels of oestrogen but also by a rise in FSH levels.

But Sandra's FSH levels weren't high – they were really low, and her oestrogen levels were barely detectable, which suggested that for some reason her pituitary gland was not working normally.

When she phoned for the results, I explained we needed to repeat the test. The levels were SO low I wondered if there had been a mistake. But no – the second test confirmed her pituitary gland was producing hardly any FSH or LH, and again, she had hardly any oestrogen.

The most common reason for that is being under-weight. It is nature's way of shutting down the reproductive system when the body does not have enough reserves for carrying and nurturing a foetus. But the threshold for pituitary shut-down with low weight is a BMI of around 18. Sandra's BMI was 20. So it was unlikely that her weight was to blame.

Much less commonly, the pituitary can be damaged if a mother has a major haemorrhage after childbirth, but that clearly hadn't happened to Sandra. Then another reason crossed my mind. Exercise. Way too much of it.

'Sandra?' I asked. 'This running of yours. How much are you doing?'

'Up until recently, I've been running five days a week for about ten miles each time and I've been trying to do a twenty-mile run once a week, I've found it a lot more difficult recently, though, because I've been so tired,' she said. In other words, she'd been doing a lot. Far more than I had envisaged.

Not only that, but Sandra told me that her training partner was hoping for a place in the GB team for the 2012 Olympics and that she herself had secured an 'elite athlete' start place for the next London marathon.

There are thought to be two main reasons periods stop in women who exercise hard. The first is that a lot of exercise can lead to the release of 'stress' hormones, which are similar to adrenalin. It's one of the reasons that exercise can make you feel euphoric, but the hormones can also interfere with the production of the hormones that control the menstrual cycle.

Too much exercise can also lead the body into believing it is in a 'starvation state'. When the amount of energy used up during exercise is not balanced by adequate nutrients from food, the body begins to shut down systems, like those controlling reproduction, that are not essential for survival. Eating the correct foods – and enough of them – is very important if this is to be avoided.

'What about diet? Presumably, with that amount of exercise, you're making sure you eat the right foods – lots of carbs? Have you had some special advice?'

'No, I thought I should just eat protein and lots of veg.'

And here lay the problem. Unlike her training partner, who was getting professional dietary advice from the British Athletics Association, Sandra was eating what she thought was a healthy diet, but in fact was far from it. Even with my limited knowledge of sports nutrition, I realised what she was eating was totally inadequate, bearing in mind how much exercise she was taking.

Although she was eating plenty of oily fish, fruit, veg and pulses, her diet contained very few, if any, carbohydrates, which are the best source of energy. Though there are no official guidelines, around a third of a healthy diet should come from carbohydrates, such as wholemeal bread, pasta, rice and potatoes. For women that should work out at around 180 grams a day and I calculated that Sandra's intake was barely a quarter of that. No wonder she was tired.

It was amazing she hadn't lost more weight. The part of her pituitary gland that controlled reproductive function had gone into shut-down, it turns out, because it realised her body could not support a pregnancy. It's a condition known medically as exercise-induced amenorrhoea.

I did a CT scan of Sandra's pituitary to be sure there was no structural abnormality such as a tumour, but when it came back normal it only confirmed my suspicions.

When we talked at length, it became apparent that Sandra had become addicted to exercise and became anxious and edgy if she was deprived of it. 'I even try to run before school as well as in the evenings,' she said. 'It's become a bit of a compulsion.'

I had to explain that the combination of too much exercise, low oestrogen and her inadequate diet were the reason she was feeling so tired.

'And, not only that, but you are putting your long term health at risk,' I explained. 'You are at increased risk of osteoporosis.'

'But I've been doing all that running. I thought weight-bearing exercise like that was good for bones?'

'It is, but strong bones need oestrogen as well.'

Sandra became very upset when I told her that the only way back to good health was to cut down on the amount of exercise she took and to eat a healthy diet based on the Food Standards Agency's 'Healthy Plate', a third of which was carbohydrates.

'You say I've got low hormone levels. Does that mean I'm menopausal? What about having children?' Sandra looked really worried.

'No, what has happened to you is the opposite of what happens at the menopause. After the menopause the pituitary works harder to try to stimulate the ovaries and levels of FSH and LH go up. Your pituitary has shut down because it senses your body is starving. But if you eat properly and cut down on the amount you've been doing, then it should return to normal – though, being honest, it's unlikely to happen straight away,' I warned her. 'It could take six months or more.' She looked relieved.

'Actually, I'm so tired it's difficult to exercise anyway,' she admitted. 'I was hoping you could come up with some miracle cure, but if it's going to take that long then maybe I should pull out of the marathon. I'm sure there's a waiting list for places.'

I agreed that was a sensible idea. I thought how ironic it was that I was telling one of my patients to cut down on their activity – normally I'm saying the exact opposite.

I also removed the Mirena coil at Sandra's request. 'I'm not in a relationship and I want my body to be free of synthetic hormones for a bit so I can assess what is happening when it's left to its own devices,' she said.

As expected, it was seven months before she had a period. She came in to see me, still slim but with more fullness in her cheeks, which had regained their previous healthy glow.

'Could I have a hormone test, just to see what's happening? I feel a lot better, but it would be good to have some evidence that everything is working again.'

Her eyes lit up when I confirmed that her body was returning to normal. 'Great – I can get back to my running,' she said. 'I really miss it and I'm getting flabby again.' My face must have shown the alarm I felt.

'Don't worry, I won't overdo it, I promise. There is a middle way. I've just got to find it and discover what my body can cope with without going into shut-down mode. I've also had some advice from my friend's dietician. I've realised if I'm going to exercise I have to adjust what I'm eating.'

Several months later, it was time for my annual masochistic ritual – the London to Brighton bike ride to raise money for the British Heart Foundation. I padded my bottom to minimise post-ride agony, did some stretches and took to the saddle. I was pleased with my effort but, once again, bloody Ditchling Beacon defeated me. I stood on the pedals, willed myself forward and then angrily dismounted, treating myself to a rant, in between taking great gulps of air.

'Hi,' said a voice.

I turned round and saw Sandra following me up the hill pushing her bike, too.

'Well hello, you,' I said. 'Last time I saw you here you vanished in a cloud of dust, making me feel hellishly demoralised and jealous.'

'This time I'm walking up this horrible hill,' said Sandra. 'I don't have anything to prove. As you know, Doctor Leonard, pushing my body beyond its limits made me so ill that I don't want to go there again. This is my middle way and I'm glad I found it before I inflicted permanent damage on myself.'

We got to the top and admired the view over the Downs together.

Sandra said wistfully, 'This may be my last ride for a bit so I'm making the most of it. Now that my ovaries are working again I've regained my libido. I didn't realise it but all that exercise had taken away my sex drive. Now I've found a really wonderful man and we've started to talk about babies . . .'